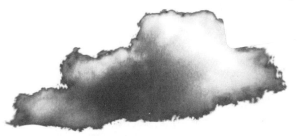

Essentials *of* Acceptance and Commitment Therapy

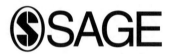

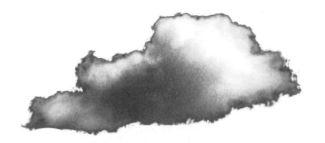

Essentials *of* Acceptance and Commitment Therapy

Sonja V. Batten

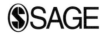

Los Angeles | London | New Delhi
Singapore | Washington DC

SAGE Publications Ltd
1 Oliver's Yard
55 City Road
London EC1Y 1SP

SAGE Publications Inc.
2455 Teller Road
Thousand Oaks, California 91320

SAGE Publications India Pvt Ltd
B 1/I 1 Mohan Cooperative Industrial Area
Mathura Road
New Delhi 110 044

SAGE Publications Asia-Pacific Pte Ltd
33 Pekin Street #02-01
Far East Square
Singapore 048763

Library of Congress Control Number: 2010934666

British Library Cataloguing in Publication data

A catalogue record for this book is available from the British Library

ISBN 978-1-84920-167-4
ISBN 978-1-84920-168-1 (pbk)

Typeset by C&M Digitals (P) Ltd, Chennai, India
Printed in Great Britain by MPG Books Group, Bodmin, Cornwall
Printed on paper from sustainable resources

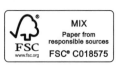

Contents

About the Author   vi
Praise for the Book   vii
Acknowledgements   ix

1   The ACT Conceptual Framework   1

2   The ACT Therapeutic Stance   9

3   Moving from Control to Willingness   18

4   Reducing the Hold of Language   28

5   Contacting the Present Moment   37

6   Identifying a Consistent Self-Perspective   47

7   Clarifying Individual Life Values   56

8   Building a Life through Committed Action   66

9   ACT for Anxiety   75

10   ACT for Depression   85

11   ACT for Substance Use and Addictive Disorders   95

12   Special Considerations in Applying ACT   105

References   116

Index   124

About the Author

Sonja V. Batten is a clinical psychologist who works on national mental health policy for the United States Department of Veterans Affairs (VA). She is also an Adjunct Associate Professor of Psychiatry in the Georgetown University School of Medicine and the Uniformed Services University of the Health Sciences School of Medicine. Dr Batten has extensive experience in acceptance-based psychotherapies, traumatic stress, substance abuse and women's health. She completed an NIMH-sponsored postdoctoral fellowship in traumatic stress at VA's National Center for PTSD. She also received specialty training in interpersonal violence treatment and research at the National Crime Victims Center of the Medical University of South Carolina. Dr Batten earned her doctorate in clinical psychology from the University of Nevada Reno, where she received multiple fellowship and dissertation awards. It was during this time that she was involved with intensive ACT clinical training and research initiatives with Dr Steve Hayes. For her undergraduate training, she attended the University of Georgia on a Foundation Fellowship and graduated first in her class. She has received multiple professional honours, including an award for Outstanding Contributions by an Early Career Psychologist to Psychology in Service to the Public. Dr Batten is also an active researcher, with an extensive international record of ACT trainings, professional presentations and publications.

Praise for the Book

'Dr Batten's world-wide reputation as an expert ACT trainer shines through in this thorough, practical and clearly written book. Her deep understanding and long experience with ACT has allowed her to produce an insightful clinical guide that those developing their ACT skills will find essential. Dr Batten presents the key ACT concepts in a way that makes them easy to understand and apply therapeutically. I have no doubt that this book will serve as a key ACT text throughout the UK and Europe.'
Professor Frank W. Bond, PhD, Head of Department, Department of Psychology, Goldsmiths, University of London, UK

'This is the best introductory guide to acceptance and commitment therapy (ACT) that I have seen. Both the theory and techniques of the ACT model of psychotherapy are often counterintuitive and confusing, even to experienced therapists. Many existing books on ACT delve into thorny theoretical issues that are only fully appreciated by those already familiar with the model, and that leave those without a thorough grounding scratching their heads in bewilderment. This book fills an important gap. Batten nicely distills the essence of ACT's core ideas in this lucid, highly accessible book. This book will be required reading for my doctoral students in clinical psychology, and I highly recommend it to any clinician seeking a clear introductory treatment to this groundbreaking work.'
James D. Herbert, PhD, Professor of Psychology; Associate Dean for Research and Graduate Education; Director, Anxiety Treatment and Research Program, Drexel University, Philadelphia, USA

'If you are looking for a clear, nuanced, and intensely practical introduction to ACT, then start with this book. Sonja has been living and breathing this work for a very long time and it shows on every page. Guided by her gentle hand, you'll be offered a unique perspective on the thinking processes that underlie effective ACT work and come away with a deeper appreciation of ACT itself. I consider this book an essential read for anyone serious about learning ACT. I am already planning to use this book as a teaching tool with my graduate students and those I supervise in clinical training.'
John P. Forsyth, PhD, Professor and Director of the Anxiety Disorders Research Program at the University at Albany, SUNY, New York, USA; and author of Acceptance and Commitment Therapy for Anxiety Disorders, The Mindfulness & Acceptance Workbook for Anxiety *and* Your Life on Purpose

'This book is a must for clinicians who are interested in learning about ACT. It is well written, practical, therapist friendly and very well organized. It provides therapists with practical guidance that can be used in clinical situations. It could easily be used as a textbook to support ACT training and supervision.'
Dr Kirk Strosahl, Psychologist, Central Washington Family Medicine, Yakima, Washington, USA

'A concise and accessible guide to Acceptance and Commitment Therapy for practitioners interested in learning about this innovative and clinically powerful approach to psychotherapy. Dr Batten draws on her extensive experience as a clinician, supervisor and trainer, to provide readers with the solid foundation they need to engage in case conceptualization and treatment planning from an ACT perspective. Her inclusion of key concepts, key terms and points for review and reflection make this an outstanding text for graduate-level trainees.'
Dr Susan M. Orsillo, Professor and Director of Clinical Training, Suffolk University, Boston, USA

Acknowledgements

Thank you to the amazing mentors I have had through the years, who have provided me with strength, guidance and opportunity: Steve Hayes, Toni Zeiss, Sue Orsillo, Victoria Follette, Paula Schnurr and many others. Without you, I could never have grown so much in acceptance of life as it is, been willing to take on those things that are important to me and had the courage to take such leaps in the direction of my values. To my colleagues at the VA Maryland Health Care System: I will always cherish our work together to develop programmes that would measure up to the amazing veterans whom we had the privilege to serve. Endless gratitude goes to all of my clients over the years and my beautiful colleagues in the ACT community, who have each taught me so much. To my amazing friends around the world: thank you for your unflagging love and support. Herzlichen Dank to my mother, Marlen, whose faith in me has never once faltered. And to my father, Wes, who once wrote to me: 'I hope that you will be able to find things in your life which are meaningful enough to *you* that you can put forth your best efforts to bring them to fruition'. Looking back, it is no coincidence that the ACT model has such resonance for me.

1

The ACT Conceptual Framework

┌───┐

| Key Concepts |

- Some techniques in ACT may be familiar to therapists from other traditions; it is the contextual behavioural theory that ties ACT together to make it unique.
- The focus within ACT is pragmatic – the emphasis is on what works for a particular person to move toward a valued life.
- From an ACT perspective, much of what is seen as psychopathology in other systems can be conceptualized as resulting from experiential avoidance.

└───┘

Acceptance and Commitment Therapy (pronounced as the word 'ACT') is an innovative behavioural therapy designed to help individuals reduce unnecessary suffering and move forward with building lives that they value. Although ACT has been in development since the early 1980s, most current ACT practitioners have become familiar with the treatment model since the year 2000 and thus see it as a new treatment. Developed originally in the United States, ACT books and trainings are now available in multiple languages and around the world. The goal of this text is to provide a practical introduction to the essentials of ACT that can be utilized as a supplement in psychotherapy training courses, or used by practitioners to reinforce ACT concepts and basic skills before or after attending an ACT workshop or training.

Revolutionary not just for the specific techniques or strategies that are incorporated into the treatment, ACT takes the pragmatic principles of a contextual perspective, along with the commitment to empirical support that is the cornerstone of evidence-based practice, and combines those philosophical assumptions with an existential and experiential sensibility. It is beyond the scope of the current text to address the core philosophy that underlies ACT in great detail. Those who are interested in an analysis of the theoretical underpinnings of this work are referred to the texts listed in the Further Readings section at the end of this chapter (see especially Hayes et al., 1999, 2001). This introductory chapter will provide a very basic overview of those theoretical principles, as well as a guide to the concepts to be covered in the rest of the text. Because the ACT model proposes that the processes at the core of problematic behaviour are common to all humans, the client and the ACT therapist are seen as being on the same level in the therapeutic relationship. Special considerations regarding the therapeutic stance in ACT will be addressed in Chapter 2.

The model upon which ACT is based can be described as having six primary areas of focus: Acceptance, Defusion, Contact with the Present Moment, Self-as-Context, Values and Committed Action. In successful ACT treatment, the therapist and client work together using these processes for the purpose of enhancing psychological flexibility and improving the client's life. It is important to note that the experienced ACT therapist will work flexibly with all six of these processes throughout treatment – sometimes using all six in one session alone. However, for the purpose of clarity in this text, these six processes will be presented sequentially (in Chapters 3 to 8). In fact, some ACT treatment protocols would have the therapist focus on these six processes in the order in which they occur in this text, and there is good theoretical reason to do so in many cases. However, there are as yet no data to suggest that these processes must be approached in a specific sequence, and many experienced ACT therapists will work through these areas flexibly over the course of treatment and depending on the client's presentation.

It is important to note that the ACT clinician does not simply move flexibly from one therapeutic target to the next simply based on moment-to-moment whim. The early part of therapy with any ACT client is devoted to a functional analysis – determining the environmental influences on the client's behaviour. How is ineffective behaviour being reinforced or strengthened, and effective behaviour being punished or weakened in a client's life, such that the person's life is not full of the things that he or she values? From an ACT perspective, there are several potential processes that are likely candidates for contributing to a client's ineffective behaviour, and awareness of these processes is used for hypothesis generation and to guide the development of a fundamental case conceptualization and treatment plan. Although multiple processes have been identified as potentially contributing to ineffective behaviour in the ACT model, such as weak self-knowledge, attachment to the conceptualized self, lack of values clarity and persistent inaction, impulsivity or avoidance (Bach and Moran, 2008), this chapter will focus on two of the most pervasive problems: experiential avoidance and cognitive fusion.

EXPERIENTIAL AVOIDANCE

Experiential avoidance has been defined as a process by which individuals engage in strategies designed to alter the frequency or experience of private events, such as thoughts, feelings, memories or bodily sensations (Hayes et al., 1996), and the resulting model holds avoidance as key in the development and maintenance of a variety of psychological disorders. Although such processes may be reinforced in the short term because they result in reduced immediate distress, they are likely to cause increased symptoms and behavioural problems over time. The concept of experiential avoidance may be best demonstrated through some common examples of major classes of psychopathology as currently categorized.

For example, in what is called Panic Disorder with Agoraphobia, an individual experiences bodily sensations, thoughts and feelings that are evaluated as extremely negative (i.e. anxiety and panic attacks), and thus avoids places, situations and things that may bring on those unwanted sensations and reactions. Gradually, as the person avoids more and more situations in the service of not having to feel anxiety or experience panic, her life becomes much more constricted and 'disordered'. From an ACT approach, an important aspect of treatment would focus on helping the client to identify the problematic role of avoidance in the development and maintenance of the Panic Disorder, before then moving on to mindfulness and acceptance work to facilitate committed action in valued domains. Similar conceptualizations exist for many other problem areas, including (but by no means limited to) substance abuse, post-traumatic stress disorder (PTSD), depression and suicidal/parasuicidal behaviour.

If experiential avoidance is so pervasive and caustic, then does this mean that all avoidance is bad? Absolutely not. The ACT approach is about flexibility and adaptable patterns of behaviour. It would be an extreme overstatement to say that all forms of avoidance are bad or will lead to psychopathology. The individual who distracts himself with music or positive imagery while having his teeth drilled at the dentist is not automatically going to develop a psychological health problem. The trouble begins when avoidance is the most frequent or characteristic way that an individual chooses to deal with difficult experiences or private events (i.e. thoughts, feelings, memories, bodily sensations) or when the person does not have other, more adaptive, coping skills upon which to rely in times of stress or distress. Chapter 3 provides more information about the assessment and identification of each client's avoidant behavioural strategies.

COGNITIVE FUSION

Another core process that is believed to be relevant to problematic or dysfunctional behaviour from an ACT perspective is known as 'cognitive fusion'. As mentioned above, ACT is based on a comprehensive theory of human language and cognition, and this theoretical model is called Relational Frame Theory (RFT) (Hayes et al., 2001). RFT suggests that one of the ways in which humans are different from any other animal is in the ability to arbitrarily relate things and events to each other and in combination, and to change the way we perceive the characteristics of specific events and experiences, simply by relating them verbally to others (Hayes et al., 2006b). Through these processes, words themselves take on the properties of the things to which they refer. This can be helpful, as calling up the word 'hammer' or the image of a hammer may help us to solve a problem, even when there is not a hammer immediately present in the environment. However, it also means, for example, that when a rape survivor has thoughts about her trauma experience, it can bring up, in the present, all of the thoughts, feelings and memories associated with the original experience, even if it was many years ago. Thus, this process of 'fusion', by which verbal processes come to excessively or inappropriately influence behaviour, may lead one to behave in ways that are guided by inflexible verbal networks rather than by the direct consequences one would encounter in the environment (Hayes et al., 1999). For example, the rape survivor who is fused with the thought 'I can't trust anyone' would be encouraged to try out a variety of interpersonal behaviours to see what happens, rather than having her choices guided by the inflexible rule suggesting that people are not to be trusted. ACT treatment, then, places emphasis on helping individuals not be governed rigidly by the thoughts and rules in their head (e.g. 'I can't stand this anxiety anymore'), working instead to find ways to interact more effectively with the directly experienced world, rather than the verbally constructed one in one's 'mind'.

It is for this reason that the ACT approach includes a variety of different therapeutic tools in its clinical or applied work. If an overly dominant focus on words and verbal constructions of situations is believed to be part of the problem, then it is easy to see how trying to 'describe' solutions or other ways of dealing with problems to clients could be counterproductive. Thus, many of the core methods of working with clients involve the use of metaphors or experiential exercises that are designed to focus people on things in their direct experience or awareness. More examples of working with cognitive fusion will be provided in Chapter 4.

EMPIRICAL SUPPORT FOR ACT

Consistent with the broad model of psychopathology suggested above, ACT has been shown to be an effective treatment for a wide variety of disorders – with much broader effectiveness across diverse conditions than most treatment approaches. Several illustrative studies and literature reviews are highlighted in the text box entitled, 'Sample of Existing Evidence for ACT'. It is important to note that this is by no means an exhaustive list, and a literature search will provide the most recent data sources. However, it does provide a sense of the breadth of the evolving ACT literature, where ACT has been shown to reduce hospitalization for psychotic disorders, improve quality of life for individuals with chronic pain, increase compliance with a medical regimen for diabetes, and improve functioning across many other domains. Further information on the evidence for ACT with anxiety disorders, depression and substance abuse will be provided in Chapters 9, 10 and 11, along with practical guidance on the application of the ACT approach to these presenting problems.

SAMPLE OF EXISTING EVIDENCE FOR ACT

Literature Reviews:

Hayes, S.C., Luoma, J., Bond, F., Masuda, A. and Lillis, J. (2006) Acceptance and Commitment Therapy: model, processes, and outcomes. *Behaviour Research and Therapy,* 44: 1–25.

Ruiz, F.J. (2010) A review of Acceptance and Commitment Therapy (ACT) empirical evidence: correlational, experimental psychopathology, component and outcome studies. *International Journal of Psychology and Psychological Therapy*, 10: 125–62.

Pain:

Wicksell, R.K., Ahlqvist, J., Bring, A., Melin, L. and Olsson, G.L. (2008) Can exposure and acceptance strategies improve functioning and life satisfaction in people with chronic pain and whiplash-associated disorders (WAD)? A randomized controlled trial. *Cognitive Behaviour Therapy*, 37: 1–14.

Wicksell, R.K., Melin, L., Lekander, M. and Olsson, G.L. (2009) Evaluating the effectiveness of exposure and acceptance strategies to improve functioning and quality of life in longstanding pediatric pain – a randomized controlled trial. *Pain,* 141: 248–57.

Other Health Conditions:

Gregg, J.A., Callaghan, G.M., Hayes, S.C. and Glenn-Lawson, J.L. (2007) Improving diabetes self-management through acceptance, mindfulness, and values: a randomized controlled trial. *Journal of Consulting and Clinical Psychology*, 75: 336–43.

(Continued)

(Continued)

Lundgren, T., Dahl, J., Melin, L. and Kies, B. (2006) Evaluation of acceptance and commitment therapy for drug refractory epilepsy: a randomized controlled trial in South Africa – a pilot study. *Epilepsia*, 47: 2173–9.

Psychotic Disorders:

Bach, P.A. and Hayes, S.C. (2002) The use of Acceptance and Commitment Therapy to prevent the rehospitalization of psychotic patients: a randomized controlled trial. *Journal of Consulting and Clinical Psychology*, 70: 1129–39.

Gaudiano, B.A. and Herbert, J.D. (2006) Acute treatment of inpatients with psychotic symptoms using Acceptance and Commitment Therapy. *Behaviour Research and Therapy*, 44: 415–37.

HOW CAN ONE THERAPY BE USED FOR SUCH A VARIETY OF PROBLEMS?

For those who are more familiar with a traditional approach to psychopathology, it can be curious to imagine how one treatment approach could be used to decrease seizures in epilepsy, as well as improve smoking cessation rates. ACT is also regularly used with anxiety and depressive disorders. Because ACT practitioners focus on the cross-cutting, functional processes that are believed to underlie many different manifestations of problematic behaviour, rather than simply on the overt form or topography of the behaviour, the most important issue is not necessarily a diagnostic category, but the patterns of behaviour that are hindering a client's successful living. In fact, many ACT-related studies have not only shown that ACT is comparable to or more effective than traditional approaches, but they also suggest that ACT works through different processes than other treatments, such as Cognitive Behaviour Therapy (CBT) (Hayes et al., 2006b).

The extremely high rates of comorbidity among the major categories of psychopathology can then be reconceptualized as the result of cross-cutting, transdiagnostic processes, rather than as multiple, co-occurring conditions. For example, if PTSD, depression, suicidality and substance abuse can all be seen as problems resulting from excessive efforts at experiential avoidance, then the clinician facing a client with these four comorbidities does not have to decide which problem to tackle first with separate, targeted treatments, but can instead proceed with one model that addresses the shared processes among all four conditions (Batten et al., 2005). Rather than primarily focusing on decreasing symptoms, the

ACT client and therapist can together work on improving the client's overall life!

The ACT model of treatment may seem complicated or counter-intuitive at first. Most clinicians report that they entered their field in order to reduce pain and suffering in others. Thus, some clinicians express scepticism when they first encounter an approach that explicitly states that it is not focused on reducing symptoms. It takes time and effort to understand the nuances in the ACT approach that suggest that pain is a natural part of living, *and* that there are things that we can do to reduce unnecessary suffering and improve quality of life. In the end, only the empirical evidence should be the final determinant of whether ACT is an approach worth learning and implementing for a given therapist. Chapter 12 provides the interested reader with suggestions about how to begin to implement ACT, growing in adherence and competence, while watching the evidence base expand to provide more comprehensive data on the promise and limitations of an ACT approach. (Please note: his and her, he and she are used interchangeably throughout this text.)

Summary

As will be demonstrated throughout this text, on its surface, Acceptance and Commitment Therapy may share formal characteristics with several other treatment approaches. However, it is based on a contextual behavioural theoretical model that focuses on processes that are common to all people, such as experiential avoidance and cognitive fusion, rather than seeing problematic behaviour patterns as the result of psychopathology. For this reason, ACT has broad applicability across a variety of presenting conditions, as is supported by the empirical literature. The pragmatic focus of ACT is on working with individuals to build lives that they value, rather than on simply reducing symptoms.

Key Terms

Cognitive Fusion: a process by which verbal processes come to excessively or inappropriately influence behaviour. Fusion may lead one to behave in ways that are guided by inflexible verbal rules, rather than by the direct contingencies and consequences one would encounter in the environment.

Experiential Avoidance: a process in which individuals engage in strategies designed to alter the frequency or experience of private events, such as thoughts, feelings, memories or bodily sensations. Such avoidance may be effective in the short term but is proposed to lead to longer-term problems in functioning if it is the primary method a person uses to deal with difficult situations or private events.

Points for Review and Reflection

- Describe two ways in which the focus of ACT differs from other therapies.
- Which clients do you think would be best suited to ACT therapy?
- How might you explore whether a person's use of avoidance is problematic or not? When were the last two times you used avoidance to deal with an experience or situation?

Further Reading

Harris, R. (2009) *ACT Made Simple*. Oakland, CA: New Harbinger Publications.

Hayes, S.C. and Smith, S. (2005) *Get Out of Your Mind and Into Your life: The New Acceptance and Commitment Therapy*. Oakland, CA: New Harbinger Publications.

Hayes, S.C., Barnes-Holmes, D. and Roche, B. (eds) (2001) *Relational Frame Theory: A Post-Skinnerian Account of Human Language and Cognition*. New York: Plenum Press.

Hayes, S.C., Strosahl, K.D. and Wilson, K.G. (1999) *Acceptance and Commitment Therapy: An Experiential Approach to Behaviour Change*. New York: Guilford Press.

Hayes, S.C., Wilson, K.G., Gifford, E.V., Follette, V.M. and Strosahl, K. (1996) Experiential avoidance and behavioural disorders: a functional dimensional approach to diagnosis and treatment. *Journal of Consulting and Clinical Psychology*, 64: 1152–68.

2

The ACT Therapeutic Stance

Key Concepts

- In ACT, a strong therapeutic relationship is seen as necessary, but not sufficient, for effecting clinical change.
- From this therapeutic stance, the therapist does not present him or herself as the expert, but rather a fellow human being who demonstrates non-judgemental acceptance for the client.
- Although the therapist works from an equal, collaborative perspective, appropriate boundaries are still maintained to ensure the primacy of the client's needs.

Whether clearly articulated or not, all traditional psychotherapies are conducted within the context of a therapeutic relationship. However, different therapeutic approaches vary in the extent to which this relationship is seen as central or ancillary to the actual work of therapy, even though it has significant impact on the outcomes of treatment across therapeutic paradigms (Lambert and Barley, 2002). Further, most treatment manuals assert the importance of a therapeutic relationship but do not detail which therapist qualities or behaviours lead to a beneficial relationship (Norcross, 2002). Within the ACT model, the development of a consistent and collaborative therapeutic relationship is considered of central importance, because it is this relationship that provides the context for the work that will be done in therapy. This chapter is thus positioned at the beginning of this text, so that the interventions that are described throughout the book can be understood within the appropriate framework. Although a strong therapeutic relationship is considered fundamental from an ACT perspective, it is not seen as sufficient to effect the necessary clinical change for the majority of presenting problems and thus should be viewed as the context within which all ACT interventions occur.

THE THERAPIST IS NOT THE EXPERT

In order to conduct ACT competently and sensitively, the therapist must strive to foster an environment in which the therapist and client are seen as being equals, on the same level, rather than having the therapist in an expert or 'one-up' position. ACT therapists are encouraged to always stay present with the awareness that they are themselves 'in the same boat' as their clients. Because the processes that lead to human suffering and problems in living are seen as universal human experiences, rather than pathological processes only experienced by those who need to come for treatment, it is assumed that therapists themselves also struggle with problems such as avoidance, fusion and lack of values clarity. The therapist must be willing to acknowledge that he is a human who struggles too – just with different content. Thus, he should also be able to apply ACT principles to his own experiences, in order to respond consistently and coherently with the model and to form an authentic relationship. If the therapist does not apply the concepts he teaches his clients to his own life, both in and out of session, then there will be a lack of genuineness in the therapeutic interactions that will stifle the development of a full and open therapeutic relationship.

Some clients will welcome this egalitarian, mutual approach and will experience the relationship as inherently validating and empowering. Others will feel initially uncomfortable with a therapist who does not represent himself as having all the answers, wondering why they should come see a therapist if he is not going to tell them how to fix their problems. Still others will assume that the therapist has reached notable levels of personal and professional achievement and thus could not truly understand the depths of the clients' struggles. In all of these cases, it can be helpful for the therapist to share his approach to his role in the therapeutic relationship:

Therapist: I want to be clear that I don't pretend to come to this with all of the answers. I could never truly know what it has been like to live through your experiences, and so I can't assume that I know exactly which way we should go as we move forward. You're the one who is the expert in the specific challenges that you have faced and you're the only one who can know what is most important to you in your life. But what I'm rather good at is helping people who are stuck get unstuck. So, what I'm hoping is that if you and I put our respective expertise together, maybe we can jointly determine how to move your life forward. Is that something you'd be willing to work toward together?

Such an approach is useful not only as a way to set the stage for the type of relationship that will be fostered during ACT, but also as a grounded way to assure the client who has been through exceptionally difficult or unique circumstances that the therapist will never pretend to know exactly what the client has been through. The assumption that therapist and client are 'in the same boat' does not mean that all experiences or types of suffering are equivalent, and the therapist must be careful not to imply that he truly 'understands' what it is like to be the survivor of torture, the war veteran, the parent who has lost a child, and so forth – because even if the therapist has been through similar circumstances topographically, the individual experience is still different. Any suggestion to the contrary is likely to be experienced as invalidating by the client. With sensitivity, the therapist can share that it is not the case that he is 'put together' compared to the client who is 'broken', but that they are both humans who struggle and who have felt pain in different ways. The therapist can then suggest that they work together from this place of mutuality:

> *Therapist*: Imagine for a moment that you're riding a bicycle up a very steep, dangerous mountain. And you come to me for help as you navigate and work your way up this mountain. If we're successful, I may be able to coach you on taking a more efficient route or avoiding a giant boulder in your path. But I want to be clear – if I am able to give you input that is useful as you ride your way up that mountain, it is not because I'm standing at the top of the mountain, having already surmounted it myself. It's because I'm on another mountain, just across the valley, working to overcome my own challenges – the distance across the valley gives me perspective on your situation and may hopefully assist you in your own successful navigation. [The therapist may draw two very rudimentary mountains and an intervening valley to demonstrate for the client the importance of perspective and how everyone is climbing his own mountain.]

Over time, experienced ACT therapists find a way to balance the straightforward acknowledgement that they do not have all the answers with the demonstration of sufficient confidence in the process that the client doesn't run from the therapy room, afraid that the therapist doesn't have enough experience to know what he is doing. This is a confidence that comes from the assumption that the therapist and client can work together through to a meaningful solution, rather than a confidence that the therapist knows exactly how to 'cure' or 'help' the broken client.

Observers often note that this very level therapeutic relationship comes across in a way that is quite different from other approaches. Consistent with codes of professional ethics that acknowledge the inherent power differential between client and therapist, ACT therapists recognize that simply by asking for help, clients enter therapy from a position of significant vulnerability. By openly acknowledging the therapist's own values about working with the client, the therapist opens up to her own vulnerability, allowing the intimacy of the therapeutic work to be established on a level field (Wilson and Sandoz, 2008). This grounded therapeutic relationship is an essential component of the practice of ACT and is stressed throughout ACT supervision and training (for more on contextual behavioural supervision, see Batten and Santanello, 2009; Follette and Batten, 2000). This open approach also gives the therapist frequent opportunities to mindfully learn from her experiences with each client.

BUILDING THE THERAPEUTIC RELATIONSHIP IN ACT

Although personal therapeutic styles vary from therapist to therapist, the prototypical relationship in ACT is characterized by openness, acceptance, respect, caring and warmth. The therapeutic relationship is used as a vehicle to model the type of relationship the client can have with her own private events. For example, when the therapist does not react with alarm or judgement to a socially unacceptable thought that the client shares, or responds irreverently when the client describes some piece of difficult content, he models that what the client is experiencing is not the enemy, it is the struggle against it that's harmful. Thus, when the therapeutic relationship is coherent and consistent with ACT principles, it allows for another way to reinforce the messages of acceptance, letting go of judgement and moving forward in the service of one's values that underlie the entire ACT model.

By demonstrating transparency and honesty throughout treatment, the therapist can help the client to build trust in the relationship. This is especially important for individuals who have been harmed or invalidated by others. Many clients, especially those who grew up in unpredictable environments, have learned to be especially skilled at reading the emotional reactions of others. Thus, trying to hide a strong response on the part of the therapist, pretending that all is well when the therapist has actually had a difficult day personally, or trying to appear that the therapist always has the answers can all serve an avoidant function and do not contribute to the ACT therapeutic environment. Instead, by sharing an honest (but never mean-spirited) emotional response or by acknowledging that the therapist himself is confused, the therapist can model openness, sitting mindfully with uncertainty and complexity, and can demonstrate how to work through toward possible alternatives in challenging situations. Making these sometimes bold therapeutic moves shows radical respect for the client in ways that simple words cannot.

A genuine sense of respect for the client's experiences, strengths and wholeness as a person is vital in ACT. The ACT therapist begins from the assumption that the client already has what he or she needs to move forward and does not try to rescue the client from the difficulty and challenge of growth. Many times, when we want to comfort someone or relieve them from their pain, it is because it makes us uncomfortable to see those we care about in distress. However, reassurance or rescuing is generally not in the client's best interest. The metaphor of the butterfly working to emerge from the cocoon applies here. Although it may seem that one is helping the butterfly by assisting it with emerging from the cocoon, it is only through the strenuous effort of exiting the cocoon on its own that the butterfly gains the strength it needs in order to fly and thrive in the world. The ACT therapist thus does not rescue his clients, but instead stands with them as they face the challenges that are in front of them. The ACT therapist also demonstrates radical respect for the client's values. This means that the therapist must truly accept that only his clients can choose how they wish to live their lives. The issue is the workability of individual choices based on the client's value system, not the therapist's own opinions.

It is only when this relationship has been established, based on acceptance, openness and respect, that the ACT therapist can truly engage in the more nuanced and challenging aspects of the therapy. For example, many ACT therapists use irreverence and humour throughout treatment. In fact, such irreverent responses can provide an opportunity to practise defusion and flexibility in real time. However, if the therapist responds irreverently or with a humorous quip to the client's personal content, without first developing a respectful, genuine relationship, the results can be extremely hurtful to the client and destructive to the therapeutic process. Even with some of the more challenging exercises in ACT, it is important that a strong therapeutic relationship has first been established, so that the client can trust that the therapist truly has her best interests in mind.

WORKING THROUGH CHALLENGING SITUATIONS IN THE THERAPEUTIC RELATIONSHIP

Even once a genuine, consistent therapeutic relationship has been established, situations will still arise that may lead to challenging interactions between therapist and client. This eventuality provides one reason that it is important for the therapist to practise mindful awareness throughout therapy, so that such situations can be promptly identified and dealt with in a way that is helpful and consistent with the ACT model. For example, if the therapist senses that there is some sort of problem or disconnect in the therapeutic relationship, he should bring the issue up in a straightforward manner, not simply avoid approaching the topic because the resulting conversation may be difficult.

In fact, the types of problems that may come up in the therapeutic context are relevant for many clients' presenting concerns, as individuals frequently report problems with relationships, intimacy or interpersonal functioning when they present for treatment. Fortunately, the therapeutic relationship can often create a context in which both effective and ineffective behaviours can be evoked. In these situations, the ACT therapeutic approach would be very consistent with the model described in Functional Analytic Psychotherapy (FAP) (Kohlenberg and Tsai, 2007). The FAP approach is based on the assumption that the therapist's emotional responses to a client are likely to be similar to the responses that are evoked in others in the client's natural environment. In response, the therapist can share his genuine reactions to the client's behaviour and thus help to shape more effective responses within the client's interpersonal repertoire through natural consequences. Avoidance of these types of potentially difficult conversations can rob the client of an opportunity to learn how his behaviour affects others positively and negatively.

Similarly, ineffective interpersonal behaviour on the part of the therapist is also likely to be present at some point over the course of therapy. The client should be encouraged to openly bring up such situations with the therapist, so that the therapeutic relationship can be repaired. In such cases, the ACT therapist endeavours to respond non-defensively and to acknowledge if he has made mistakes or done something that has hurt his client. By approaching such situations with humility and genuineness, and working immediately to repair the relationship, the therapist demonstrates that he knows that he, too, is human and prone to imperfection. If handled well, such situations can provide an important learning experience for both therapist and client.

Another situation in which the therapist may have a strong emotional reaction is when the client reaches a barrier in treatment or does not follow through with an action to which he or she had committed. Such situations can bring up natural feelings of frustration, sadness and disappointment for the therapist who cares deeply for his client's well-being. These situations can provide an important opportunity for the therapist to get in touch with his own struggles and remember how difficult it can be to move forward at times – even when it may seem to someone else that it should be easy to follow through. Reminders of the therapist's own humanity can be very important in these moments, so that he can respond from a place of kindness and compassion rather than frustration.

Newcomers to the ACT approach sometimes worry that this type of mutual, open therapeutic relationship might lead to inappropriate therapeutic boundaries. In fact, the boundaries of the therapeutic relationship in ACT are natural and linked to workability, rather than being entirely rule-governed. However, workability is always defined by what is in the best interest of the client, which includes compliance at all times with relevant ethical guidelines. It is true that the ACT therapist may regularly make self-disclosures during sessions if he believes that to do so could be important for building the therapeutic relationship or helping the client move forward more effectively. This does not mean that the therapist uses the therapeutic relationship to garner support for his own struggles or to help him feel more comfortable. Certainly, the ACT therapist might be more likely than therapists from other theoretical models to share that a recent interaction with the client led him to feel sad, if he thought that such feedback could assist the client with a therapeutic target. However, the decision is less clear when disclosing information about the therapist's life or history. In ACT, there would be no de facto rule, for example, that would prohibit a therapist from sharing with a client who is a trauma survivor that the therapist had also experienced a traumatic event as a child. However, the decision to do so would not be simple. Before making such a disclosure, the ACT therapist would be expected to seek consultation or supervision and to think carefully through the function that such a disclosure would be expected to serve. The therapist would need to examine whether the urge to disclose this information is truly for the potential benefit of the client, or is instead in the service of helping the therapist to feel more connected to the client or less alone himself.

CONSIDERATIONS FOR THE THERAPEUTIC RELATIONSHIP IN ACT

Although ACT can at times be an intensely emotional therapeutic approach, especially once the client has broken through the barriers of avoidance into willingness and acceptance, ACT therapists do not focus on emotion solely for emotion's sake. The topographical display of emotion is irrelevant to the principles and practices of ACT. Crying or other types of emotional experiencing are only consistent with the ACT model if they serve to move the person closer to her values and goals. Conversely, although much of the language used to describe ACT concepts and metaphors can come across as intellectual and 'heady', it is important that the ACT therapist steer away from intellectualizing in the session and point out this unhelpful process when either the therapist or client are becoming overly intellectual or analytical in a way that does not serve the needs of the moment.

In situations where a client is unable to label her own emotions (often associated with growing up in an inconsistent, invalidating environment), the therapist can use her empathy and connectedness to suggest possible emotions the client may be feeling. However, these should always be expressed as hypotheses (e.g. 'Would it be accurate to say that you're feeling angry right now?' or 'If I were in your situation, I think I would feel quite disappointed. Do you think that you're feeling at all disappointed?'), so that the client can disagree openly if the labels do not fit. In the context of a strong therapeutic connection, the skilled therapist can work with the client over time to gradually move from alexithymia (the inability to express feelings with words) to awareness to acceptance of the full spectrum of emotional experience.

As a final note, it is important to recognize that the central role of the therapeutic relationship as described here does not preclude the effectiveness of learning ACT principles through bibliotherapy or online methods of training. In fact, promising data are emerging that suggest that many of the concepts of ACT can be effectively learned and implemented in ways other than in a traditional interpersonal context. This chapter has simply described the characteristics of the therapeutic relationship that are posited to be most helpful when ACT is delivered in interpersonal psychotherapy settings.

Summary

The therapeutic relationship in ACT serves as a model for the relationship the client is working toward developing with respect to his own personal experiences and private events. By showing openness, acceptance and respect, the ACT therapist builds a collaborative approach in which client and therapist work together to bring the client closer to a life that she values. Although more egalitarian than some approaches to therapy, ACT therapists still recognize appropriate and ethical boundaries within the therapeutic relationship, in a manner that is consistent with function and workability.

Points for Review and Reflection

- Describe three characteristics of an effective therapeutic relationship in ACT.
- Why wouldn't an ACT therapist choose to frame himself as an 'expert' to a new client?
- Describe two ways that an ACT therapist shows respect for his clients.
- As an ACT therapist, how might you think through whether you should share an emotional response you are having in a session with your client?

Further Reading

Batten, S.V. and Santanello, A.P. (2009) A contextual behavioural approach to the role of emotion in psychotherapy supervision. *Training and Education in Professional Psychology*, 3: 148–56.

(Continued)

(Continued)

Follette, V.M. and Batten, S.V. (2000) The role of emotion in psychotherapy supervision: a contextual behavioural analysis. *Cognitive and Behavioural Practice*, 7(3): 306–12.

Kohlenberg, R.J. and Tsai, M. (2007) *Functional Analytic Psychotherapy: Creating Intense and Curative Therapeutic Relationships*. New York: Springer.

Wilson, K.G. and Dufrene, T. (2008) *Mindfulness for Two: An Acceptance and Commitment Therapy Approach to Mindfulness in Psychotherapy*. Oakland, CA: New Harbinger Publications.

Wilson, K.G. and Sandoz, E.K. (2008) Mindfulness, values and therapeutic relationship in Acceptance and Commitment Therapy. In S.F. Hick and T. Bien (eds), *Mindfulness and the Therapeutic Relationship* (pp. 89–106). New York: Guilford Press.

3

Moving from Control to Willingness

Key Concepts

- The ACT therapist works with his client to identify the role that excessive internal control efforts have played in the development and maintenance of the client's presenting problems.
- The ACT perspective maintains that it is not that the client has not worked hard enough, tried hard enough or had enough willpower; it is that purposeful control of thoughts and feelings is a problematic strategy for effective living.
- For clients to move toward psychological flexibility and workable life choices, they may need to work on increasing willingness to experience the full range of private events, in the service of valued life directions.

From an ACT perspective, many of the problems in living that bring clients to therapy are related to an unwillingness to experience their own thoughts, feelings, memories and other private events. Although it is natural to avoid things that one finds to be unpleasant or aversive, pain, anxiety, loss and disappointment are all part of the human experience and cannot truly be avoided in any long-term manner. One of the ways that the ACT therapist helps clients to move toward psychological flexibility is by introducing the possibility that this focus on internal control may itself be part of the problem that has led the individual to seek treatment. The concept is that by reducing control over internal events, clients are freed up to exert more control over their lives.

INTRODUCING THIS APPROACH TO TREATMENT

As described in Chapter 2, it is very important for the ACT therapist to work to build rapport and trust with the client by being direct, respectful and forthright. This applies throughout the therapy, but certainly is essential in the first several therapeutic interactions. At the beginning of treatment, the ACT therapist garners true informed consent from the client. This type of informed consent includes not simply the standard information about limits of confidentiality and possible treatment alternatives. In addition, the ACT therapist attempts to describe what is different about this treatment, so that the client has a better idea of the proposed approach:

> *Therapist*: Before we really begin with the main work of this treatment, I'd like to tell you a little bit more about it. You said that you've been in therapy before, and so I need to let you know that this approach is somewhat different from what you may have encountered with other therapists. In the type of therapy that I do, the focus is not on helping you to feel *better*, but instead to *feel* better. I propose that if we can work on helping you to find a different way of responding when difficult thoughts and feelings arise, this may be more effective in helping you to move forward with your life than if we just focused on helping you to feel less sadness and anxiety.In fact, I think it's likely that here, at first, those symptoms of sadness and anxiety may sometimes go up, and sometimes go down, like waves in the ocean. What I'm suggesting is that we commit to a piece of work together for however long seems OK to you at first (3 sessions, 6 sessions, 10 sessions, etc.), and that at that time we take a look to see how things are going. My request at that point will be that we assess whether we're making progress not by how you happen to be feeling in that moment – because we know those waves of feelings will vary from day to day and moment to moment – but by whether you have the sense that things are moving forward and that what we're working on together has the potential to make a difference in how you live your life.

Some clients may have had enough experience with other modes of therapy to be ready to try something new. Others may have had the types of life experiences or exposure to spiritual traditions that have opened them to an awareness that pain is part of life. For those individuals, they may feel immediately validated by a therapist who does not suggest that the removal of psychological distress is the ideal end state. However, for other clients who are more caught up in the struggle with their own private experiences, the idea that one might not need to change or reduce unpleasant private events in order to move forward with life may seem nonsensical or misguided. For these clients, it can be useful to begin therapy with a stage that is called (among therapists, generally not between therapist and client) 'Creative Hopelessness'.

CREATIVE HOPELESSNESS

By the time that clients come to therapy, they are frequently disappointed and frustrated and may have little hope that their lives can actually change. They might feel that they have tried everything possible to deal with their depression, their anxiety and their ineffective habits. The ACT therapist approaches this point from a new angle. What if it is not the case that the client has not tried hard enough, worked hard enough, been smart enough or demonstrated enough willpower to change? The ACT therapist introduces this concept and suggests another explanation: perhaps the client has simply been applying a strategy to solve a problem that cannot work for that purpose.

Therapist: I hear you saying that you feel completely stuck right now, unsure that there will ever be a way out of your current struggles. You even used the word 'hopeless' a few minutes ago. And I think there may, in fact, be a degree of hopelessness here – but not in the same way that you mean it.

Client: Well, if you're saying that this is hopeless, then why should I be here?

Therapist: Let's be clear. I'm not saying that you are hopeless, or even that the situation is hopeless. What I am suggesting is that maybe the strategies that you have been using so far are hopeless. It seems to me that you have been working very hard at trying to solve this situation and change the way things are for quite some time now. And what if it's not the case that these strategies just haven't worked *yet*? Instead, what if it's the case that these strategies *can't* work to solve this particular problem? [pause] Sometimes I think it's helpful to have an image to capture what I'm trying to say. I'd like you to imagine that there's a patch of quicksand in the woods, and some sort of animal – maybe a deer – lopes along and falls into the quicksand. What is that deer's first instinct going to be? To struggle like mad to try to climb its way out! [Therapist mimes this struggle with flailing arms and legs.] And we all know from watching movies or cartoons what happens when you try to struggle your way out of quicksand, right?

Client: You go deeper and deeper down in the sand.

Therapist: Right! So, instead, we know from watching those same movies that we're supposed to do something counter-intuitive if we have the unlucky circumstance of falling into quicksand ...

Client: Lie flat and stay still.

Therapist: Exactly. You're supposed to stop struggling, spread yourself out and try to get in as much surface area contact with the quicksand as possible – at least as an initial step until you figure out what else to do. But the first thing is to stop struggling and just get in contact with

> the stuff that you're struggling with. I guess I'm suggesting that maybe
> it's not that you haven't been trying hard enough to deal with your
> current situation – it's just that sometimes we have to realize that
> we're in the quicksand, so that we can stop struggling long enough to
> try something else.

Clients generally respond well to these sorts of metaphors. Having an image or a story to refer back to can serve as a kind of shorthand between the client and therapist throughout treatment. The metaphor of struggling in quicksand is just one way of helping the client to see that sometimes the next step is counter-intuitive. Many other metaphors have been created that suggest this same point (e.g. Person in a Hole, Tug of War with a Monster; see Hayes et al., 1999); the important thing is to find a way of describing the process to which the client can relate (it is even better if the therapist can identify something from the client's own experience that fits). In the process of Creative Hopelessness, the clinical goal is to work with the client to get into experiential contact with the awareness that the current tools or strategies have not worked and likely will not work. If the client can recognize, for example, that digging with a shovel is a rather hopeless way of getting oneself out of a hole (shovels are there to dig holes deeper!), then this opens up all manner of other creative strategies that can be attempted instead, once the client puts down the shovel.

GIVING THE STRUGGLE A NAME

If the client is willing to consider that the struggle itself may be part of the problem, then it becomes important to move the discussion from the metaphorical into the personal. As described in Chapter 1, ACT theorists and researchers have posited that experiential avoidance plays an important role in many different clinical presentations, including depression, anxiety disorders and substance abuse, to name a few. Regardless of the specific diagnoses that can be given in these instances, it is argued that excessive attempts to avoid or control private events (e.g. thoughts, feelings, memories, bodily sensations) are a key functional problem. For the concepts presented in the creative hopelessness phase of treatment to have resonance for the individual, the therapist must help the client to identify which strategies have and have not been working in the client's life.

This process is generally begun by asking the client to share what he has tried so far in an effort to deal with the problems that have brought him to treatment. Frequently, those answers will include things like: drinking alcohol, a variety of modes of distraction, retreating to sleep, overanalysing things or taking medication. Depending on how long the therapist and client have for this process, they could work together to develop an exhaustive list, or just to identify a few primary strategies that the client has used. The goal is to have enough of a sample to be able to identify a theme among the majority of the items. A more detailed example will be provided in Chapter 11, to include illustrative language for eliciting the items on the list, as well as drawing out a theme that ties many of the strategies together.

If the client is presenting with problems that are hypothesized to have an experiential control component, then many times the cohesive theme can be summarized as 'control' or 'avoidance'. It is important to note, however, that the specific words used are not what are important. There is no 'right' answer to be found in this process. In fact, there may be idiosyncratic reasons not to focus on certain words with certain clients. For example, the abuse survivor by definition has experienced a loss of control. Thus, trying to explain to her that the therapist will be working with her to reduce unnecessary aspects of control may bring up a number of unhelpful associations that can temporarily derail the work of that session. The key step for the therapist is to find a way of speaking that resonates for the client and that helps the client to put a label on what her own version of struggling in quicksand is.

As each of these strategies is identified, and again when reviewing the full list, the therapist will ask the client some variant of the question, 'And how has that worked for you so far?' The therapist must ask this question without judgement or preconceived assumptions of what the answer should be. Of course, the therapist likely holds the hypothesis that the majority of these efforts have not worked, or the client would not be sitting in the therapy office. However, the therapist must always be open to the individual's own experience, and some of the efforts identified may well have worked to a certain point or in a certain context. If the therapist appears to be fishing for a specific answer from the client, some clients will automatically reply with the opposite of the expected response. On the other hand, if the therapist explores the workability of the client's choices and strategies with a genuine curiosity, compassion and openness, client and therapist will together have the best possibility of confronting the true functionality of a variety of ways of responding to the client's problems. At the end of the session in which these concepts are discussed, the therapist will often give a homework assignment to practise awareness of these processes until the next session:

> *Therapist:* OK, so we've discussed a lot of things this week about some of your patterns that seem to keep you stuck, just like struggling to get out of quicksand would get you more and more mired in the sand. And we identified that, for you, one way to look at what that struggle is can be boiled down to 'control'; that a lot of those things that haven't seemed to work for you, at their core, are about trying to control your own experiences – either by holding on to those thoughts and feelings that you want to keep, or by avoiding or pushing away those that are difficult or painful. And I don't think it would be fair for me to simply ask you to change without giving you some alternatives. So, for this week, I'd just like to ask you if you'd be willing to do one thing. I would

like you to see if you can just be aware and notice when you are doing some of those things that we labelled as 'control'. See if you can try to just be aware of how often during the week you're struggling in that quicksand. Next week, we'll start to look at some alternative ways of responding. But remember that the first thing to do when you're in quicksand is just to notice where you are and let go of the struggle. That's what I'd like you to experiment with this week.

IF CONTROL IS SUCH A PROBLEM, THEN WHY DO WE ENGAGE IN IT?

There are likely to be a wide variety of individual reasons that a person would engage in experiential control or avoidance strategies; Hayes and colleagues (1999) have categorized these reasons into four major domains. First, we often learn to control our private experiences (or at least the expression thereof), because we watch parents and other influences model emotional control as we grow up, and from the outside, it looks like these efforts work (e.g. seeing a parent regularly having an alcoholic drink to deal with stressful situations). Second, we are often directly instructed by others to engage in such control efforts (e.g. 'stop crying or I'll give you something to cry about', 'be a big boy/girl'). Third, control strategies generally work very well in the external world, and thus it seems natural to apply these strategies to private events as well; for example, if one wants to get rid of an unwanted object in one's environment, usually a small amount of problem solving will lead to success. Fourth, control even seems to work sometimes in the internal world with thoughts and feelings – at least in the short term (e.g. through distraction or reassurance). Because humans (as all animals) are much more likely to be affected by short-term, rather than long-term, consequences, it makes perfect sense that experiential control strategies would be so ubiquitous!

WILLINGNESS AS THE ALTERNATIVE

If we are to understand control and avoidance as largely ineffective strategies implemented in efforts to change, decrease or remove unwanted private experiences, then the ACT therapist must be able to provide potential alternatives for the client to practise when such thoughts, feelings and memories arise. Within ACT, the primary alternative to control is described as willingness or acceptance (hence the term 'Acceptance' in the name of the therapy). In short, willingness is seen as a process in which an individual can choose to open up and experience the full range of private experiences, without having to change or defend against them. The heart of ACT involves repeatedly working with the client to be willing to experience whatever private events arise, in the service of being able to more successfully move forward with his life. To be willing to have difficult thoughts and feelings is not the same as wanting those experiences. It is also unlike indulging or attempting to hold on to any given experience. Willingness also has a different quality to tolerating or putting up with difficult experiences. Note that ACT does not suggest that individuals should accept or tolerate aversive or harmful external circumstances that they actually have the power to change. Instead, willingness entails a posture and way of responding to one's own internal experiences that is open, undefended and flexible.

It can be rather difficult to simply describe these different ways of responding to one's own private events using verbal instructions alone. Just as one can't learn to ride a bicycle simply by listening to someone describe the mechanical steps involved in pedalling, steering and balancing, ACT therapists recognize that verbal descriptions alone will seldom be enough to convey what is meant by choosing to be 'willing' to experience the full range of thoughts, feelings, etc. Several willingness exercises can be found in the original ACT text (Hayes et al., 1999), and therapists can make up an infinite number of additional exercises, once they themselves understand the concepts to be conveyed. Sometimes these concepts can be best presented as physical metaphors:

> *Therapist*: So, I know that I've been saying that there's an alternative to this struggle and proposing that it might be this thing I'm calling 'willingness'. But I'm guessing it may not be entirely clear what I mean when I say that.
>
> *Client*: That's true. I mean, I understand the word, and I can use it in a sentence, but I really don't have any idea what you're actually asking me to do when I feel like I'm about to have a panic attack.
>
> *Therapist*: OK, well, I wonder if you'd be willing to do an exercise with me, so that I can demonstrate what I'm talking about. [Client agrees.] What I've got here is a stack of these small notecards, and what I'd like for us to do for a few minutes is to write down the types of thoughts, feelings and bodily sensations that come up when you start to feel that high anxiety. [Therapist and client spend several minutes writing individual items each on a notecard, such as 'Difficulty breathing', 'Knot in my stomach', 'Panic!', 'I can't take this anymore!'] So, now we've got this stack of cards, and on each of them, we've written something that shows up for you alongside the anxiety that you've generally tried to struggle against and get rid of. Is that right?
>
> *Client*: Yes. It makes me a little bit anxious just looking at that stack of cards right now.
>
> *Therapist*: OK, cool.

After creating the stack of personalized cards together, the therapist then asks the client if she'd be willing to try relating to the cards in some different ways, just to see what it is like. The therapist explains that he will be gently tossing these cards in the client's direction and suggests that she can choose various ways of responding. For example, he might first suggest that she try to fight these experiences as they show up. So, he announces the content on each card as he carefully tosses them one by one toward her. In response, the client uses her arms to bat the cards away as they come near her. They go through the stack of cards that way, and the client is asked how that experience was for her. Then, they pick up the cards again, and the therapist suggests that they try the exercise again, but with a different mode of responding. For example, the second time through, the client might be asked to try to ignore or hide from the different experiences by holding her hands up in front of her eyes, so that she can't see the cards. The therapist then initiates the same process by announcing the content on each card as he carefully tosses them in her direction. Some of the cards bounce off, while others may land in her lap and stay there. The client is again asked to describe her experience. Finally, the therapist asks if they can do the exercise one more time – this time, the client sits openly with her arms and hands facing up in her lap, signifying that she is welcoming whatever lands there without having to fight it, hide from it or defend against it. As with the second posture, some of the cards land in her lap, while others bounce off on to the floor.

> *Therapist:* So, I guess I'm curious to hear what you noticed in this exercise. How were those three postures or ways of responding different for you?
>
> *Client:* Well, the first one was sort of stressful and tiring, but at least I felt like I was doing something. And with the second one, I felt somewhat protected by having my hands in front of my face – I could pretend for part of the time that nothing was happening.
>
> *Therapist:* That's really interesting. And what about the third time?
>
> *Client:* Well, the third time was kind of scary at first, because I didn't know exactly what was going to happen. And I still didn't like what was on those cards coming over to me. But after a little while, it got a little more peaceful, once I realized that the cards themselves really couldn't hurt me. It was actually sort of interesting watching to see which ones were going to bounce off on to the floor and which ones were going to land in my lap and stay there for a while.

The therapist can do much during the processing of this exercise. Obviously, the primary objective of this physical metaphor is to demonstrate the functional differences between control, avoidance and willingness, and much more can be done to elaborate on those points. It is important, though, that the therapist also use this as an opportunity to point to the differences in workability between these three strategies. Using examples of potentially valued activities in the client's life, the client can be asked from which of these postures the client would best be able to hold a conversation with a friend, study for a class or engage in other valued actions while the cards are coming forward. It is essential that this link be drawn to show the unworkability of avoidance and control – although these strategies may work in the short term, they severely limit an individual's ability to do other important things in life while the difficult content is present.

It is also important to demonstrate through metaphors, experiential exercises and discussion that a willingness-based approach is really all or nothing. One is either open and willing, or not. One could choose to practise willingness only in certain contexts or for a limited amount of time – nobody is 100 per cent willing all the time (especially when willingness skills are first being learned and practised). However, one cannot limit willingness based on the intensity of the experiences. For example, if a client indicates that she can try willingness with her anxiety only to a certain point, because she certainly couldn't be willing to experience the full range of private events during a panic attack, the ACT therapist helps the client to see that willingness 'to a point' is not really willingness. To relate to some of the previous metaphors described, this would be like spreading out and making contact in quicksand only to a certain point, saying that if she got too much deeper in the sand, she'd have to start struggling again. Or in the notecard exercise, it would be similar to starting with the open, non-defended posture, but then starting to bat away or hide from certain cards that held content considered especially aversive. One is either fully willing, or one is not willing.

CONSIDERATIONS FOR MOVING FROM CONTROL TO WILLINGNESS

These messages of moving toward willingness can be very scary or challenging to contemplate, especially for the client who has had a very difficult history, or who has very intense private experiences. It is important that the therapist remind the client that this is a choice that only the client can make. Over time, the client's life will provide the data to indicate whether or not a willing approach facilitates more effective living. Willingness is not the same as wallowing around in difficult content. The therapist is not suggesting that the client slog around in a nasty, filthy swamp just for its own sake. The therapist helps the client to look up ahead and see that there is a life worth living on the other side of the swamp, and that they can move through the swamp together. The hard work of willingness becomes meaningful and is dignified because it is in the service of something important – building a life worth living, rather than remaining stuck.

Summary

ACT therapists work with clients to identify strategies that the client has already tried in order to deal with her presenting problems. The workability of each of these strategies is assessed; if a particular strategy has not been successful, then the therapist and client should reasonably focus their efforts elsewhere. From an ACT perspective, these unsuccessful strategies can often be conceptualized as serving a control or avoidance function. In these cases,

(Continued)

(Continued)

the therapist will introduce as an alternative the process of willingness to experience the full range of private experiences, in order to bring the client closer to a valued life.

Key Terms

Creative Hopelessness: a phase of ACT treatment in which the therapist works with the client to identify those strategies (often those that centre on attempts to avoid or control unwanted private events) that have not been working effectively for the client. Through this process, the therapist hopes to illuminate the hopelessness of such control strategies, so that the therapist and client can creatively determine other alternatives.

Willingness: a process in which an individual chooses to experience his own private events without defence, in the service of moving forward with a valued life. This process is differentiated from tolerating, wanting or wallowing in these experiences.

Points for Review and Reflection

- Bring to mind a specific issue, emotion or problem that you've been struggling with for an extended period. Identify at least five ways that you have attempted to deal with or change this problem. Is there a theme that ties the majority of those strategies together?
- Experiential control is a ubiquitous process. Provide specific examples of how a person's early experience would lead him to practice experiential avoidance and control, even though it might have adverse, long-term consequences.
- Identify a specific time in your life when you chose to be willing to experience difficult thoughts, feelings or bodily sensations, not because you wanted them, but because doing so was in the service of something that was important to you.

Further Reading

Harris, R. (2009) *ACT Made Simple*. Oakland, CA: New Harbinger Publications.

Hayes, S.C. and Smith, S. (2005) *Get Out of Your Mind and Into Your Life: The New Acceptance and Commitment Therapy*. Oakland, CA: New Harbinger Publications.

Hayes, S.C., Strosahl, K.D. and Wilson, K.G. (1999) *Acceptance and Commitment Therapy: An Experiential Approach to Behaviour Change*. New York: Guilford Press.

4

Reducing the Hold of Language

| Key Concepts |

- The human ability to use language is exceptionally powerful; however, it can bring with it a cost when the products of one's mind are taken too literally.
- Defusion processes are used in ACT to help clients respond in a different, more flexible way to their own cognitive content.
- The goal of defusion is not to reduce the distress associated with difficult thoughts, feelings and images, but to bring about behaviour that is more consistent with the client's values and the workability of such behaviour in his life.

Language is so automatic for verbally capable humans that often we don't even notice that the sometimes arbitrary and reflexive thoughts that go through our minds are just another example of 'languaging'. Because the words and thoughts that we experience happen so seemingly naturally, we often treat them as if they are real or true. Our cultural context reinforces our response to language, such that if we have a thought that says, 'I like ABC' or 'I can't do XYZ', we will most likely behave in a way that is consistent with that cognitive content. In many cases, this ability to think and act based on verbal content ('put that dish in the oven for 30 minutes to cook it fully') can be extremely useful and is responsible for much of what humans have been able to accomplish over the past several thousands of years. However, from an ACT perspective, this verbal ability is also seen as having unexpected negative consequences. This chapter will introduce ways of working therapeutically to break down the cognitive fusion described in Chapter 1.

THE LIMITS OF LANGUAGE

Because of the human ability to use language, words take on the actual characteristics and functions of the things to which they refer. This is why in the notecard exercise in Chapter 3, just looking at the notecards with difficult content written on them made the client slightly nervous. The same thing can happen for anyone when just thinking about a difficult experience brings up associated emotions, behaviours and urges. Of course, an ACT therapist wouldn't want to take away this function by which all manner of characteristics and stimulus properties are called up by language alone – this ability is very adaptive in many ways. However, ACT practitioners work to add to these functions to disrupt some of the processes that cause problems when cognitive content is taken too literally.

The process known as 'cognitive fusion' is thought to occur when the verbal characteristics of events (how we judge, evaluate and think about things) are more prominent in a person's experience than the natural consequences and contingencies that occur in the person's actual environment and inform whether or not a behaviour is workable and adaptive (Bach and Moran, 2008). Not all fusion is problematic – if you're following instructions to get to somewhere that you've never been before, then being able to act based on verbal content (e.g. directions that someone told you) rather than direct experience is functional. However, if a person treats verbal content literally, such as the thought 'I'm not really welcome at that party tomorrow night', when feeling anxious about being in a new social situation, it can keep the person from engaging with the environment and being shaped by the direct contingencies of interacting with others who may in fact have enjoyed spending time with this person. Thus, the goal of defusion processes (also known as 'deliteralization' in some texts) in ACT is to undermine the problematic dominance of verbal processes over the natural consequences in life that would otherwise shape behaviour adaptively.

One of the problems with excessively aligning behaviour with cognitive content is that much of what is generated by our 'minds' is not particularly useful. If it were all useful, then we would not have to consider fusion as a problematic process. However, much of what 'pops' into our minds at any given moment is simply automatic because of our learning history, and the remainder is often arbitrary and not particularly meaningful. So, when we treat the content of our thoughts as true and sacrosanct, it makes it more likely that our behaviour will be similarly arbitrary and automatic.

The mind's ability to generate negative content has an adaptive function, because it allows people to predict and respond proactively to potentially dangerous scenarios. Thousands of years ago, the ability for the mind to call up the image and characteristics of a predator or other danger that was not currently present could increase the individual's ability to engage in protective behaviours that would improve her chances of survival. However, such immediate dangers are no longer a part of many people's day-to-day experience. Even so, our minds seem at times to continue this process in overtime – predicting danger and negativity where there is none, with correspondingly narrow and self-protective behaviour.

Furthermore, although the mind is very useful in a number of domains, it also overestimates the utility of language and thoughts as being all-powerful. To demonstrate some of the limits of language, an ACT therapist works with the client to first recognize that there is a distinction between the description of something and the thing described. For example, one could read a book about Antarctica and learn all sorts of important facts about the country. One could even learn to recognize digitally vivid pictures of Antarctica that look extremely realistic. However, none of those representations or symbols would actually be able to approach the full experience of standing at the South Pole with high winds and all of the associated sights and sensations. Within ACT, it is often said that words seem on the surface as if they are just as solid as the things they describe. For example, although one could describe a bicycle down to very precise detail, one cannot actually ride the description of a bicycle, regardless of how specifically it is described. Words can also appear as if they are just as useful as one's direct experience. However, as referenced in Chapter 3, one cannot teach someone how to ride a bicycle through words alone. The bicycle trainer might be able to suggest the main factors that require attention during the activity, but as many people can remember from the first time they learned to ride a bicycle, there are no words that can truly convey all the myriad of movements and micro-balancing that must be done in order to ride successfully.

THE PROCESS OF DEFUSION

The concepts described above are used as background for the work of defusion in ACT. Because language and cognitive fusion are, by definition, human phenomena, defusion is a skill that is universally relevant in ACT. All individuals are expected to be able to benefit from the ability to gain some distance from their cognitive content, rather than responding automatically to thoughts as if they are literal truths. For example, the individual with a long history of interpersonal disappointments may never stop having the thought, 'No one can love me', arise from time to time. However, if he is able to successfully defuse from that thought, then the thought does not have to lead to socially isolative behaviours and worsening of depression. Similarly, the individual with a history of agoraphobia may have all manner of thoughts about leaving home and going to new places (e.g. 'I just can't go out today'). Within ACT, this individual would learn not to try to rid herself of this thought and reassure herself of her safety, but instead to see that thought for what it is – the arbitrary and automatic product of her mind's functioning that does not need to be followed as if it were truth.

Several metaphors can be used to demonstrate what it would be like to defuse from cognitive content, rather than waiting for difficult thoughts to go away before being able to move forward in one's life. The therapist can refer back to the swamp metaphor described at the end of Chapter 3:

> It's as if when you're traversing through the swamp, a voice keeps calling out negative things to you: 'You'll never be successful! You might as well quit now!' You can stop and respond to the voice – challenging it, telling it to stop and covering your ears, or you can notice that it's there and keep moving through the swamp regardless of what that voice is saying, because you know that life is waiting for you on the other shore.

Another image that can be helpful is one from television or movies where an individual has a little angel on one shoulder, and a little devil on the other shoulder. In such a scene, the person's attention is batted back and forth as the angel and the devil throw out content to support their ways of looking at the world. Imagine that the character in this show is able to recognize that he may never be able to get rid of that little devil and little angel, but he does have full control over whether he engages with them or not. The angel and devil don't have to go away before he can continue walking and moving forward in his life in directions that are important to him.

In addition to such metaphors, many brief experiential exercises are also used to provide clients with the direct experience of defusing from the content of their thoughts. The most well recognized of these ACT exercises may be the 'Milk, Milk, Milk' exercise (Hayes et al., 1999), which was adapted from an exercise designed for a different function by Titchener (1916). In this exercise, the client is asked to identify the range of possible associations that are brought to mind simply by saying the word 'milk' out loud. Then, the client and therapist repeat the word over and over, quickly and loudly, for approximately 30–45 seconds. Afterward, the client is asked to describe the experience, which generally results in the literal properties of the word being broken down, and the formal properties of the word (the sound of the word as spoken) becoming more prominent. Frequently, clients report that the meaning of the word is temporarily lost and the associations with 'milk' that were previously present are now more distant. The extension of this exercise is to consider the possibility that the thoughts and other cognitive content that one struggles with on a regular basis may not have any more substance or truth than 'milk, milk, milk, milk, milk'.

With an exercise such as 'Milk, Milk, Milk', the ACT therapist seeks not to invalidate or minimize the difficult thoughts and beliefs that a client holds by reducing them to a series of sounds, but rather to help the client respond differently when those thoughts arise. This can be distinguished from some approaches within the cognitive or cognitive behavioural therapy traditions. In ACT, the goal is not to change the content of thoughts or replace negative content with more accurate content. Instead, the ACT therapist works to show clients how to put more space between themselves and their thoughts. In addition to the 'Milk, Milk, Milk' exercise, the therapist may also work with the client to experiment with different ways of hearing and saying these thoughts. The therapist might recommend that the client practise saying difficult words or phrases in different voices (high, low, with an accent), at different rates of repetition (quick, slow), in different song styles, or even in the voice of a political leader that the client does not respect (e.g. 'And if you could hear that thought in the voice of so-and-so, would you take it nearly as seriously?').

Within the discussion of defusion, it is also useful to come back to the notecard exercise described in Chapter 3. If one views this exercise from a different angle, it should be apparent that the exercise also serves a clear defusion function. Writing the thoughts down on cards allows some distance from the information that the mind is producing. Seeing them written down as an external entity allows the client to look 'at' rather than 'through' those thoughts. Depending on what is necessary in the session, the therapist and client can play around with holding the thoughts close to the face or far away, to show differences in perspective. The therapist can also give homework to walk around with the cards during the week (by placing them in one's pocket or purse, or even under a pillow at night) to see what it's like to carry around such content mindfully and still continue to move forward and live life.

Defusion is reinforced as clients increase mindfulness skills and the ability to stay in the moment, rather than getting trapped inside verbal content. By definition, many mindfulness techniques also have a defusion function. These approaches to gaining distance between one's experiences in the moment versus the content of one's mind will be highlighted in Chapter 5.

Such processes require ongoing practice. Just as our eyes adjust when we don glasses with blue lenses, and we begin to see the world through that layer of blue, forgetting that our experience is coloured by the lenses themselves, humans see the world through the filter of language and must frequently practise different ways of recognizing the influence of that lens. Defusion techniques are seen as one way to remove those blue glasses from time to time, so that individuals can experience the world more directly, even if the effect is not permanent.

WORD CHOICE AND LANGUAGE CONVENTIONS TO PROMOTE DEFUSION

Throughout ACT, the therapist also makes specific language choices to assist the client with defusion and simply being aware of her own thinking. For example, the therapist will frequently talk about what the client's 'mind' is doing. This is not because ACT therapists are Cartesians who believe that individuals have a mind that is somehow separate from the rest of the person's body, but because using the metaphor of these processes being the product of the client's 'mind' can help one to recognize the process of thinking more dispassionately and to identify why fusion with these thoughts may or may not be helpful. By keeping the referent of a sentence like, 'I'm suggesting that maybe it's the case that your mind is not your friend', as the 'mind', it can allow therapist and client to talk about some of the problematic aspects of verbal behaviour and thought without spurring the client to become defensive. Further, talking about what the 'mind' does can itself be used as a defusion technique, as long as the therapist is clear that he is speaking metaphorically, not literally.

ACT therapists frequently refer to the mind in other ways as well. For example, when a client shares an evaluation or particularly judgemental thought and seems especially fused with the content, the therapist may choose not to respond to the content, but instead respond by saying, 'You can thank your mind for that'. If there is a strong therapeutic relationship, the therapist may experiment with even more irreverent ways of pointing out the never-ending process of the mind's work. For example, when describing the incessant yammering of the mind, the therapist may also make a corresponding hand gesture of the hand opening and closing rapidly to suggest a mouth that talks and yaps on and on. If the client seems to respond well to this hand gesture once or twice, the therapist can then use it silently in future interactions as a non-verbal cue to point out to the client times when excessive fusion may be present. Further, as described in Chapter 2, the therapist is not immune to the problematic aspects of thought and language and may make this clear in the context of defusion by saying something to the effect of: 'And you know, at any given time, there are actually four of us in the room – you, me, your mind and my mind. We can't ever stop what either of our minds may choose to go on and on about while we're in here, but we can keep an eye out for when that's happening to make sure that we're not getting lost because we've gotten locked into what either of them is saying'.

Several other language conventions are also used to bring attention to the process of thinking and 'languaging'. As part of defusion, clients are taught to identify and overtly label when they are having thoughts and feelings, rather than automatically buying into those experiences. For example, a client who makes a statement like, 'I'm so anxious. I just can't take it anymore', will be asked to restate this comment as, 'I'm having the feeling of anxiety, and I'm having the thought that I can't take it anymore'. The same process can be done with bodily sensations, urges and other private experiences. The idea is that by having to slow down and label these experiences for what they are (not what they say they are), the client will, over time, learn to gain some distance from these experiences without having to fuse with or avoid them. Similarly, the therapist may work with the client to be able to label whether a given thought is a description (non-judgemental reporting on a process) or an evaluation (adds subjective judgement of good/bad, etc.). Thus, the therapist may expand 'I'm having the thought that …' to include 'I'm having the evaluation that …'. Without the ability to recognize the distinction between evaluation and description, the client may not notice the key difference between a thought such as 'I am a person' and 'I am a horrible person'. Finally, Hayes and colleagues (1999) describe another important language convention that teaches clients to replace the word 'but' with 'and'. 'And' can be seen as a word that is descriptive and allows for all possibilities, whereas 'but' cuts off options and requires reasons to be taken literally. By working with clients to use 'and' instead of 'but', the ACT therapist reinforces the idea that no thought or reason needs to be taken as the literal determinant of subsequent behaviour.

The purpose with all of these language conventions is not just to get the person to talk differently for the sake of formal change. The hope is that by adding in some of these slightly artificial processes, it can help point to what our minds do naturally. If successful, we may better see those processes for what they are and hopefully create a little bit more space between the thinker and the thoughts. When these language conventions and other defusion efforts function as designed, we can actively choose how to respond to thoughts, rather than simply reacting automatically. As with all aspects of ACT, the goal is not to reduce the level of distress associated with these thoughts or to change the form or frequency of various cognitions. The goal is flexible living and workability related to the individual's values.

CONSIDERATIONS FOR WORKING WITH DEFUSION

The therapist should be on the lookout for opportunities to practise defusion throughout the course of therapy. Defusion can be an appropriate intervention in many circumstances. However, there are several types of content that are especially susceptible to cognitive fusion and the resulting psychological inflexibility. For example, Harris (2009) identifies six key areas where fusion may be likely to occur: Rules, Reasons, Judgements, Past, Future and Self. These categories are by no means exhaustive, and there are obviously a tremendous number of situations where fusion can be problematic (including fusing to 'positive' content). But for the beginning ACT therapist, ongoing awareness of these potential 'sticky' areas may provide a guidepost to help remind the clinician when it might be useful to be on the lookout for fusion and to implement defusion techniques.

Throughout the work of defusion, it is important to note one caveat: the therapist should be careful to avoid invalidation or minimization when using defusion techniques around difficult personal content. Defusion can absolutely be done broadly, even with some of the most painful content, and the ACT therapist must not buy into the perspective that some cognitions are so true, painful or sacrosanct that they cannot be approached in the same way that one would approach any other type of cognitive content. However, the therapist must do so carefully, sensitively and in the context of a strong therapeutic relationship. Defusion is a component of ACT where the irreverent responses discussed in Chapter 2 can be used to their full advantage. Done well, this part of ACT can be liberating, light and sometimes fun, even when dealing with very painful or challenging content. This work can model the notion that the therapist is not afraid of the client's content, even when it feels terrifying or horrifying to the client. Thus, this is another example of where the therapeutic relationship can itself be used to model consistency with the principles of ACT that are being taught in the session.

Summary

If defusion processes are successful, the therapist and client will be able to begin placing thoughts in a context of mindful awareness, rather than a context in which the content of thoughts are taken as literal truth. There are an infinite number of exercises or strategies that can be implemented to assist the client in learning how to defuse from challenging cognitive content; the goal of all of these exercises and language conventions is to help the individual gain more distance from those thoughts, so that he or she can make choices based on values and workability in the natural environment, rather than based on believing his own thoughts as 'truth' or following inflexible verbal rules.

Key Terms

Defusion (also known as deliteralization): any therapeutic process in ACT that serves to undermine a problematic dominance of thoughts and verbal content (vs. direct experience) over behaviour.

Literality: a context in which individuals take the content of their thoughts as literal truths, and thus act in ways that are consistent with that cognitive

(Continued)

(Continued)

content. (This can be contrasted with a context of mindful awareness, in which thoughts are seen as automatic, sometimes arbitrary products of language and relational responding that may or may not be used to guide behaviour.)

Points for Review and Reflection

- Describe two differences between how a traditional psychotherapy model, such as CBT, would approach difficult cognitions, and how ACT would approach the same cognitions using defusion. What are the differences in the strategies used, and the goals of the interventions?
- Which aspects of implementing defusion strategies or techniques do you think might be challenging for a new ACT therapist?
- What is the purpose of the many potential language conventions used by an ACT therapist who is working on defusion processes with a client?
- Choose a difficult thought with which you regularly struggle. Try out three of the defusion exercises suggested in this chapter. What do you notice about your experience of this thought during each of the exercises?

Further Reading

Bach, P.A. and Moran, D.J. (2008) *ACT in Practice: Case Conceptualization in Acceptance and Commitment Therapy*. Oakland, CA: New Harbinger Publications.

Harris, R. (2009) *ACT Made Simple*. Oakland, CA: New Harbinger Publications.

Hayes, S.C. and Smith, S. (2005) *Get Out of Your Mind and Into Your Life: The New Acceptance and Commitment Therapy*. Oakland, CA: New Harbinger Publications.

Hayes, S.C., Strosahl, K.D. and Wilson, K.G. (1999) *Acceptance and Commitment Therapy: An Experiential Approach to Behaviour Change*. New York: Guilford Press.

5

Contacting the Present Moment

Key Concepts
- Although it can be useful to reflect on past events and plan for the future, many individuals who present for psychotherapy focus excessively on the past or an imagined future, rather than living their lives in the here and now.
- Within the ACT model, being in contact with the present moment is essential for defusion, acceptance, experiencing the self as the context for one's experiences and living consistently with one's values.
- Mindful awareness can be cultivated through a variety of formal and informal exercises and practices.

From a contextual behavioural perspective, there is no moment other than the present moment. However, because of the uniquely human ability to use language and respond relationally, we can organize our behaviour and choices around events in the past or things we imagine in a verbally constructed future (even if we've never before directly experienced the types of things we're imagining). This ability to focus attention on time perspectives other than the present moment is certainly adaptive in many ways, including allowing us to plan behaviour that is consistent with valued directions. Nevertheless, if our behaviour is primarily determined by these verbal constructions, it reduces our ability to behave with psychological flexibility and respond appropriately to the natural consequences in our immediate environment. Although not part of any specific diagnostic nomenclature, many of the problems that bring individuals to treatment have at their core some type of problem with remaining in the here and now. For example, lack of contact with the present moment can lead to behaviours that range from daydreaming to ruminating about the past or future to dissociation at the most extreme end of the spectrum; furthermore, behaviours such as substance abuse or purposeful self-injury can be seen as concrete examples of the lengths to which individuals may go to become out of contact with the present moment.

Within the ACT model, contact with the present moment is important in and of itself, but also because it is directly related to each of the other five major ACT processes. None of those other processes can be fully engaged from any perspective other than within mindful awareness of the present. For example, values that are identified without full contact with the present are likely to be more influenced by verbal rules or the expectations of others. Similarly, willingness and acceptance cannot be practised from any perspective other than the here and now.

So, what does it mean to be in contact with the present or to practise mindfulness? Mindfulness can be described as participatory, non-judgemental observation of whatever is occurring in the present (Gunaratana, 1992). The definition by Kabat-Zinn (1994) adds the specification that there is a purposeful quality to mindfulness – simply being swept away by the moment is not the same as being mindfully aware. Within the practice of ACT, contact with the present moment, or 'being present', can be described as having a vital, creative and connected quality (Luoma et al., 2007). Being mindful and aware as we go through life, making large and small choices, is the primary antidote to behaviour that may otherwise feel as if it happens on 'autopilot'.

THE PRACTICE OF MINDFUL AWARENESS OF THE PRESENT

Given the fundamental importance of connecting with the here-and-now experience, it is important to ensure that clients in ACT treatment are able to discriminate when they are or are not practising awareness of the present moment. Although one may be able to understand conceptually what is meant by the words 'contacting the present moment', it is not always as clear exactly how to go about doing so. Because it is difficult to explain such an experiential process solely through verbal instructions, it can be useful to train the skill of mindfulness more explicitly through practice both in and outside of the therapy session.

One common misconception is that practising mindfulness is the same thing as meditation. It is important to note that a mindfulness practice does not require formal meditation; however, some forms of meditation are certainly consistent with a present-moment focus. Any activity in which an individual can bring purposeful, non-judgemental attention to the experience builds the capacity to stay in the present moment. Over time, the idea is that individuals can learn how to be mindful of, rather than reactive to, even the most challenging thoughts, feelings and bod-ily sensations. In order to build that capacity, it can be helpful to work with the client on multiple modes of practising mindfulness and contact with the present moment. These practices can take a myriad number of forms – somatic/sensory, imaginal or even physical. Dozens of these practices are outlined in other texts (see Hanh, 1976; Kabat-Zinn, 1994 for many, varied examples). To provide a brief introduction to the breadth of such practices, there are below brief scripts for several ACT-consistent exercises that can be utilized both in and out of the ACT therapy session. These selected exercises are simply examples of the different modes of practice and should not be seen in any way as a com-prehensive list. The scripts below are not meant to be read aloud verba-tim and can be modified and adapted based on the needs of the client and the particular moment. Further, when actually using one of these scripts, the therapist would insert many pauses between statements, allowing time to notice and practise the points described and to adjust the pacing for each particular client. Following each exercise, the thera-pist may choose to spend either a short or a longer time processing the experience with the client, depending on the case conceptualization and needs in that session.

Body Focused Mindfulness

'I'd like us to take just a few moments to try to connect with our current experience. And so I'd ask you to start by getting comfortable in your chair in a position where you can sit for a few minutes. Go ahead and either close your eyes, or just gently look down at a spot on the floor and let your eyes become unfocused. As you take a few deep breaths, see if you can begin to become aware of the sensation of breathing in and out. And then begin to notice the sensation of your body touching the chair. Try to notice all of the places where your body touches the chair – and once you've identified all of those spots, imagine that you have a piece of chalk and you're able to move that piece of chalk and actually trace around all of those places where your body touches the chair. [Allow time for the client to do this imaginally.] And when you have that out-line complete, imagine that it is filled in, so that you can see the full shape of all the places where you are in contact with the chair. Now notice the sensations of your feet touching the floor. See if you can actu-ally experience the sensation of gravity holding your feet to the floor.

Next, we'll move to noticing the range of sensations that are going on within your body right now. Let's start to move up from your feet into your lower legs and knees. Notice whatever you can about your muscles and the feeling of your clothes on your skin. Moving up your legs and to your hips, just be mindful of any sensations that you encounter. Remember, as you continue moving up through your lower back and abdomen, that your job right now is not to categorize or evaluate any of those sensations – just non-judgementally bring each one into awareness and then move on to the next one. If you're identifying any places where you have discomfort or tension, simply breathe in and see if you can imagine the breath swirling around in that area for a moment before you mindfully breathe out. As you move up through your belly and chest into your upper back, see if you can become aware of sensations that you do not usually notice. Next, begin to shift your awareness into your neck and throat and allow yourself to contact whatever sensations are present. Finally, moving up to your head and face, notice the feeling of your scalp and skin, as well as any unexpected areas of tension that you were previously unaware of. Now, we will simply sit quietly for a few minutes, and I'll ask you to just see if you can stay in contact with the experience of what you notice as you sit inside your body. If you start to be pulled away by thoughts or evaluations, just notice that, and come back to the sensations inside your physical self.'

Breathing Mindfulness

'So, this time as we work on becoming centred and grounded in the moment, I'd like to ask you to focus for a few minutes on your breathing. As you become grounded in your chair and ready to begin the exercise, go ahead and shift your attention to your breathing. You might start by taking a few deep breaths, noticing how far you can comfortably expand your lungs and chest as you breathe in, and how your muscles and the air interact as you breathe out. Go ahead and take a few deep breaths. [Pause while the client does so.] Now you can return to just breathing as you normally would – not too shallow, not too deep. Notice the range of sensations that happen in your nose, mouth, throat and chest as you breathe in, as the air swirls around in your lungs, and then rises back up through your throat and out again. Just spend a little time becoming aware of these sensations as you breathe in and out, in and out. Now shift your attention from your body to instead pay attention to the air itself. For example, see if you can notice that the air you breathe out is a little warmer than it was just a few seconds ago as you were breathing in. Now, I'll be quiet for a few minutes and allow you to take in the totality of the experience of breathing, recognizing that this is an opportunity to be mindful of an experience with many layers that is going on all the time, whether you choose to be aware of it or not.'

Clouds in the Sky

'Now that we've gotten grounded and centred here in the moment, I'd like to see if we can practise becoming mindful today of the range of thoughts that might go through our minds at any given time. So, if you're willing, I'd like you to try to imagine that you're looking up into the sky. It's a bright blue sky, and you become aware for just a moment of that exact shade of blue. As you look up into the sky, you begin to see large, fluffy clouds moving slowly from one edge of the sky across to the other side. And they keep coming, one after another, moving across the sky. Just watch that sequence of events for a moment. And what I'd like to ask you to do now is to begin to become aware of whatever thoughts are popping into your head from moment to moment. And as you begin to mindfully become aware of those thoughts, I'd like you to picture taking each thought as it arises and placing it on a cloud and watching it go by. Just take each thought as it comes up, place it on a cloud and let it float to the other side of the sky and out of your field of vision. You might choose to represent each thought on the cloud with a word, phrase or image – the form does not matter, just the process. And if you find yourself becoming distracted from the exercise or thinking that you can't do this, then as soon as you notice that, just take that thought and place *it* on a cloud, watch it go by and return to the process. You may have to do this over and over again, and that's OK. There's no finish line. It's just an opportunity to practise being mindful of your thoughts and to detach from them, rather than becoming hooked on them or buying into them.'

It is important to note that this same exercise can be done with different imagery, such as leaves on a stream, boxes on a conveyer belt, train cars on a train track or little toy soldiers walking in a line holding signs. The therapist can work over time to find the imagery that may work best for each individual client. For those clients who have difficulty labelling what it is that they are feeling, more shaping by the therapist may be necessary, and the use of a list of feeling words can be very helpful.

Five Senses

An infinite number of variations of this exercise can be practised. The idea is to take an object and to cycle through mindful attention to each of the five senses in the moment with respect to that object: sight, smell, touch, taste and sound. For example, the therapist might have a piece of fruit or chocolate and ask the client to interact with the piece of food and focus on each of the senses for a minute or two in turn, leaving taste for last. The same thing can be done with inanimate objects or items such as hand lotion (although one obviously might not choose to taste certain items or objects). It can also be a fun change of pace for both the client and therapist to practise mindfulness with pieces of music. For example, in a piece of music with strong instrumental characteristics, the client can be asked to switch between purposeful awareness of the different instruments that are playing, recognizing that the others still go on, even when the focus is just on one part. Similarly, with a piece of music that has sung lyrics, the client can be asked to attempt to focus on the sound of the vocals, rather than the meaning of the lyrics. This can both be a fun exercise, as well as one that points to the need for defusion skills, due to the automatic processes by which our minds focus on the meanings of words to the exclusion of their other characteristics.

Mindfulness on the Rocks

This model comes from an exercise practised in clinical trainings and therapy groups by Andrew Santanello and Sonja Batten. At its core, it begins with a 'five senses' mindfulness exercise, but with an ever-changing stimulus. This exercise is one that can be especially productive to practice in a group therapy setting, as each of the individuals in the group will have an assortment of both shared and individual experiences. To begin with, each individual in the group is allowed to pick a piece of ice from a bowl as it is passed around the room. It is hard to identify a standard size for such a piece of ice, but a small to medium-sized piece of ice works best. As the ice is being passed around the room, the group leader explains the following:

'As you choose your piece of ice, if you are willing, all we are going to ask you to do is to place it in the palm of one of your hands and simply allow it to rest there. No need to do anything with it. Just begin to watch what happens as your hand comes into contact with the ice. At first, you are probably drawn to noticing the physical sensations of your hand as it becomes cold from the ice, and then may begin to feel numb. See if you can separate out the actual sensations from your verbal labels and then evaluations of those sensations and return to just being mindfully aware of what it feels like with the ice in your hand. Next, I'd like you to focus on what you can see. What does the surface of the ice look like? How does it reflect the light? And what can you see about the water that is beginning to pool in your hand as the ice melts?

As time goes by and the ice continues to melt, you may notice a variety of reactions going through your mind. For example, you may be feeling an urge to move your hand so that the water will spill from your hand and on to the floor. If that's the case, just notice that urge and see if you can sit with it without doing anything. Others of you may be worrying about whether it's OK to hold a piece of ice for this long or may be asking yourself why you chose such a large piece of ice. That's OK, too. Just watch those reactions and see if you can let them go and come back to the direct experience of being in contact with the ice itself. You might choose to close your eyes for a moment, and as you breathe in imagine that your breath flows in and swirls around in the area where you are having the most intense sensations or urges to move. See if you can take this as an opportunity to practise willingness, rather than avoidance or fusion with your thoughts and urges. Now look at your hand and see how your hand has been changed by its time in contact with the ice. Has it changed colour at all? If so, look at the shape of the area that may be a little redder than the rest of your hand. And, finally, as the ice finishes melting in your hand and becomes a small pool of water, see if you can watch what your mind tells you about wanting to wipe your hand off so that it will be dry. Notice those thoughts, and if you're willing, see if you can allow your hand to simply air dry.'

Mindfulness While Engaging in Activities

Another classic mode for practising mindfulness is to choose to be mindful while engaged in any type of physical activity. The beauty of this way of practising mindfulness is that one does not need to carve out a specific period of time during the day to practise and can work on refining mindfulness skills anytime and in any circumstance. For example, one can practise being mindful of the five senses, or of thoughts and feelings that arise, while washing dishes, listening to music, vacuuming the floor, travelling on the bus or train, walking down the street or when interacting with another person. The activity itself is irrelevant as far as this type of practice is concerned. Instead, what is important is the ability to truly engage in the activity, fully and without distraction, choosing to be present in that moment, over and over again. Such practice may be especially useful for those individuals who have trouble with imaginal exercises. In addition, by practising mindfulness multiple times throughout the day, and in a variety of contexts, individuals increase their ability to generalize mindfulness skills to be used in any situation.

THE ROLE OF MINDFULNESS IN ACT THERAPY

As discussed above, the ability to remain in contact with the present moment is an essential skill that provides a solid foundation from which to implement all of the components of ACT, and mindfulness practices comprise one important way of developing the ability to increase present-moment awareness. Mindfulness can thus be practised in the session either formally or informally. Some therapists may choose to begin each session with a brief mindfulness exercise to orient the client to the present and begin that day's therapeutic work. It is important to note that mindfulness exercises in sessions are not just for the direct benefit of the client. Many therapists who find themselves rushing from session to session or moving quickly from administrative activities to therapy during the day also report that it is useful for them to practise mindfulness as a way to contact the present moment and connect with the work that is there to be done with each individual client.

Other therapists may not choose to teach mindfulness through formal in-session exercises, instead using moment-to-moment awareness in a session as a way of practising mindfulness and enhancing the therapeutic work. Mindfulness can also be used in sessions when one is feeling stuck (Wilson and Dufrene, 2008). In those moments in therapy where it is not clear where to go next or when the therapist and client do not seem to be working productively together, it can be exceptionally useful to slow down and practise mindful awareness of the therapeutic process. By contacting the totality of that moment's experience of feeling stuck in such situations, therapist and client alike may be able to reconnect with the present and with each other and move forward again together. Finally, on a very practical level, therapists often come to a session with a specific plan or agenda, based on the case conceptualization and the events of previous sessions. Although having a general plan can be very valuable, it is also important to practise a present-moment focus in the session, or the therapist will likely miss important information and the ability to be flexible based on what is actually happening from moment to moment.

CONSIDERATIONS IN CONTACTING THE PRESENT MOMENT

Regardless of how successful and moving mindfulness exercises practised in the therapy session have been, simply practising present-moment awareness once per week with a therapist will not be sufficient to truly gain the capacity to be mindful in all types of situations. It is even more important that the client is able to generalize this skill to a variety of contexts. Thus, for many clients, the therapist should encourage and monitor the practice of 'real-world' mindfulness in between therapy sessions. For such generalization to be successful, the therapist should work with the client to practise mindfulness in a variety of contexts and through multiple methods (e.g. somatic, imaginal, activity-based, eyes open and eyes closed). Because there are currently no data to suggest that any one of these modalities is more effective than others, it is recommended that the therapist and client work together to find modes of practice that are most useful for that individual. Within this individualization, it is important to note that certain clients may have strong or unexpected reactions to particular types of practices. For example, clients with a physical or sexual trauma history may initially have significant difficulty with exercises that focus on the body or physical sensations. Similarly, traumatized clients who frequently engage in dissociative behaviour may dramatically lose contact with the present during closed-eyes or imaginal mindfulness practices. For these individuals, it is recommended to begin with more concrete, participatory exercises that can be accomplished with one's eyes open.

Although caveats are provided for ways to modify mindfulness exercises for some clients, this should not be taken as a suggestion that some individuals will simply not be able to connect with the present moment. What may need to start with mindfulness of relatively neutral, external things, as individuals begin to learn mindfulness and associated practices, can be built all the way up to being able to be present and mindful with even the most challenging of content, sensations or emotions. This ability to practise mindfulness is fundamental to the ability to practise acceptance and defusion and move forward with effective living that is consistent with one's values. Although there is much more to ACT than simply being mindful, without this ability to move forward from the perspective of present-moment awareness, little else will be able to be fully accomplished.

Summary

In ACT, present-moment awareness undergirds all of the work that is done between the client and therapist. Many clients have significant difficulty being in contact with the here and now, and ACT therapists can work with their clients using a variety of tools to be able to engage in non-judgemental attention to thoughts, feelings and bodily sensations. By practising these skills in and out of session, the client will be able to generalize the ability to use mindfulness skills in order to be able to sit non-reactively with a wide variety of private events, even those that are initially the most personally challenging.

Key Term

Mindfulness: a process that can be described as the purposeful, participatory, non-judgemental observation of whatever is occurring in the present. Mindfulness is often experienced as having qualities of creativity, vitality and connectedness.

Points for Review and Reflection

- What challenges can you imagine with practising present-moment awareness from the perspective of the client? And from the perspective of the therapist?
- Try for yourself three different types of mindfulness exercises. How might you adapt such exercises for use in a range of settings?
- What sort of clinical presentation might be associated with initial barriers or obstacles to being in contact with the present moment?

Further Reading

Hanh, T.N. (1976) *The Miracle of Mindfulness*. Boston, MA: Beacon.

Kabat-Zinn, J. (1994) *Wherever You Go There You Are*. New York: Hyperion.

Kabat-Zinn, J. (1990) *Full Catastrophe Living: Using the Wisdom of Your Body and Mind to Face Stress, Pain, and Illness*. New York: Dell.

Williams, M., Teasdale, J., Segal, Z. and Kabat-Zinn, J. (2007) *The Mindful Way Through Depression: Freeing Yourself From Chronic Unhappiness*. New York: Guilford Press.

Wilson, K.G. and Dufrene, T. (2008) *Mindfulness for Two: An Acceptance and Commitment Therapy Approach to Mindfulness in Psychotherapy*. Oakland, CA: New Harbinger Publications.

6

Identifying a Consistent Self-Perspective

Key Concepts

- All individuals define themselves by a variety of labels, evaluations and roles – both positive and negative; within ACT, this is known as the 'conceptualized self'.
- It is natural to see oneself from the point of view of the conceptualized self; however, inflexible and ineffective behaviour can result when one is overly attached to this perspective of self-as-content.
- The ACT model suggests several exercises and practices by which one can instead learn to experience a consistent perspective of self-as-context, wherein one is not fundamentally defined by the content of one's thoughts, feelings, evaluations or history.

From the time that children begin to use language, they are gradually taught to describe their own behaviour, preferences and experiences. This use of language is certainly adaptive, as it allows communication about needs, desires and events that have occurred in the child's life. However, because human minds are so good at evaluating and categorizing things, it is not long before the ability to describe and judge gets turned upon oneself. For example, it may develop quite naturally that a young child begins to describe himself as a 'boy', and then as a 'good boy' or 'bad boy', and then as a 'good boy/bad boy who is afraid of dogs' and on and on. Although these descriptors may initially seem simple or innocuous enough, the ACT model entails that over time, we begin to fuse with these descriptions and evaluations to such an extent that they come to have great influence over our behaviour. A resulting behavioural constriction develops as we automatically begin to align our behaviour in accordance with the self labels with which we have fused.

This set of labels and descriptions that we each have for ourselves is known within ACT as the 'conceptualized self'. It is important to note that the conceptualized self is neither good nor bad in and of itself. It is problematic only when we become overly attached to this conceptualization and truly believe that we are defined by those labels in a firm or unchanging way. For example, one person might see herself as an 'overweight, business executive, mother of three, who does not get along with her family'. Although one could look at each of these labels and try to parse out to what extent each one is 'true', it is actually not the truth of any of the labels that is important. The impact of these labels comes with how firmly the individual believes them. For example, if this individual has the evaluation 'overweight' as a defining characteristic of who she believes she is, this may lead her to decline to go to a pool party for a good friend's birthday, because she does not want to wear a bathing suit. Or, if she sees herself professionally as a business executive, this could lead to her choosing not to pursue an interest in art and photography – and so on and so on. The labels themselves are not the problem; it is the *attachment* to those labels that can keep people stuck in roles and judgements, rather than in direct experience and moving forward based on values.

When individuals recognize that they are not their content, labels or history, then they can open up to try new things, move forward and behave flexibly and effectively. Furthermore, it is not the case that only negative self-concepts can be a problem. More positive self-labels can be just as damaging if they are believed literally and function to constrain behaviour. It is not as simple as divesting from the negative aspects of the conceptualized self and increasing the number of positive self-evaluations that are believed. Rather, individuals need to be able to hold all of these labels and evaluations more lightly. Thus, one of the primary goals of ACT involves working to both defuse from these labels and verbal constructions and to attempt to find a new way of experiencing the perspective of what the 'self' is.

This work is among the most abstract within ACT. What does it mean to find another perspective by which to experience the self? And why is this distinction so important? The answers to these questions are more likely to be contacted experientially, rather than effectively described verbally. The second section of this chapter will describe several of the relevant experiential exercises and metaphors that make this distinction. At an overview level, the alternative to experiencing a sense of self that is defined by the content of one's thoughts, feelings, memories and bodily sensations is to find a 'place' in which one can connect with a transcendent sense of self that has always been present and that is safe and not determined by transient thoughts, feelings, etc. If one can identify and choose a perspective in which one's identity is not defined by the content of one's experience, then the perceived danger of experiencing difficult private events is reduced. This perspective, in which one is able to connect with a consistent sense of self that transcends thoughts, feelings and labels, is known in ACT as self-as-context.

The process of contacting this place of self-as-context requires skills of both defusion and a mindful, present-moment focus. The goal of this phase of ACT is to assist the client in distinguishing the 'person' from her 'programming'. This reinforces the work of defusion, reminding the client of the arbitrariness of much of the cognitive content that arises naturally (described in Chapter 4). If the client can learn through experience that he is not defined by his sadness, shame, anxiety or troubling memories, then maybe there is another way to relate to this internal content. In this ACT component, the therapist works with the client to connect with a different perspective – a sense of self that is not determined by thoughts, feelings or any other private experience. If there is some place from which these experiences can be safely observed, then perhaps one does not have to run from them. The ACT model proposes that there is no pain that is so great that the person cannot contact it, because no thought, feeling or memory is permanent. The only thing that abides – that is consistent – is the 'I' that provides the context from which each of these things can be observed.

SELF-AS-CONTEXT EXERCISES AND METAPHORS

Progressive Self Questions

At the most basic level, targeted interventions in the self-as-context component of ACT attempt to contrast the constantly changing content of private experiences with a consistent perspective from which one can mindfully observe this ever-changing content. For example, in a session, the therapist may ask a series of questions to illustrate the distinction between the observer and the things that are observed:

Therapist: And what can you notice in your body right now?
Client: I'm feeling tense and it's hard to breathe.
Therapist: And who's noticing that tension and shortness of breath?
Client: I don't know if I understand your question. I mean, I am. Is that what you mean?
Therapist: OK. And can you tell me a feeling you're having right now?
Client: Um, I guess I'm feeling nervous and confused.
Therapist: OK. And who's noticing those feelings of nervousness and confusion?
Client: I am. Who else would be noticing them?
Therapist: Sure. And what about thoughts? Can you share a thought you're having right now?
Client: I'm having the thought that things are never going to get better.
Therapist: OK. And who's noticing that thought, here and now?
Client: I am. But what's the point of that?

Therapist: We could go on and on with this, and we could identify an infinite number of thoughts, feelings, sensations and memories that pass across your awareness, right? Because that's what our experiences do. They come and go, come and go. And lots of times, it seems like those experiences – those thoughts, those feelings – are the problem. But what I'm trying to help you contact here is that although these experiences come and go constantly, there's a part of you there that is able to notice them. That's the part of you that you were referring to when you answered my questions by saying, 'I am'. There's a part of you that's always there, always aware of everything, and that stays safe regardless of which experiences are present. I'd suggest that we try to do some more work to go into that perspective where you're not defined by your thoughts and feelings, because I think that might give us a safer place to do this work, rather than if your whole being is determined by those ever-changing experiences, which is how your life has been going a lot of the time recently.

The Observer Exercise

A more structured and in-depth version of the Progressive Self Questions exercise is known as the Observer Exercise (a full script for this exercise can be found in Hayes et al., 1999). In this exercise, the client is guided through an imaginal exercise in which she is asked to notice her ever-changing roles, thoughts, feelings and even her physical body. As she identifies her experiences in each of these domains, she is then asked to identify who is noticing each of those experiences. She is also asked to see if she can identify this observing self-perspective across a variety of memories at different stages of her life, to demonstrate that the observing self (often described as 'the you behind your eyes, who watches and notices everything that you experience') is always there and is not fundamentally changed by any given experience. The observing self is able to dispassionately, mindfully notice the content of one's experience, without being affected by it in any fundamental way. From this perspective, one's thoughts, feelings and other experiences are not the enemy – they are simply content to be noticed by the observing self.

A House with Furniture in It

Another metaphor that can be used to demonstrate the distinction between content and the context in which the content is held is the 'House with Furniture in It' metaphor. In this metaphor, the client is encouraged to visualize a house with several rooms in it – any type of house will do. The client might first be asked to imagine that the house is empty of any furniture or decorations. However, over time, various pieces of furniture are placed in different rooms of the house. Some of these furnishings are what the client would label as 'stylish' or 'attractive'; other furnishings might be labelled by the client as 'hideous' or 'old-fashioned'. The client should be asked to imagine all manner of furniture cycling in and out of the house, over and over, while the house itself remains structurally unaltered. After doing this for a couple of minutes, the therapist can then point out to the client that although the contents of the house came and went, with both desirable and undesirable items, the fundamental nature of the house remained unchanged. The house is simply the container or context that holds all of the pieces of furniture. Similarly, the observing self can hold any type of private experience (thought, feeling, memory, etc.) that the client may have – the pieces may come and go, but the container (or context) remains stable and consistent.

A Container with Stuff in It

In a further elaboration of the House with Furniture in It metaphor, the therapist may choose to act out a similar process experientially in the session. For this exercise, the therapist will need a box or container of some sort to place on the floor between the client and therapist (an office rubbish bin works well for this purpose), as well as several tissues or disposable pieces of paper. The therapist asks the client to begin by identifying a thought, feeling or memory that he has been struggling with. A tissue is brought out to represent that difficult private experience, and the therapist may even cough or spit into the tissue to represent its perceived unpleasantness. The tissue is thrown into the container. The therapist then asks the client for a reaction to looking at the initial tissue, and the client shares a thought, feeling or urge that comes up as he thinks about that initial item. Whatever shows up next is then represented by a tissue or piece of paper, wadded up and thrown into the container. Over time, after doing this repeatedly, the bin begins to fill up with tissues and papers, until perhaps the initial tissue is no longer visible. The therapist can use this as an opportunity to reinforce concepts from earlier in treatment that it is not possible to avoid or get rid of any private events – only to add new ones on top of the old. (As is often said in ACT: 'The nervous system only works by addition, not subtraction'.) The messages of self-as-context can also be reinforced – the container itself is not changed in any meaningful way by whatever manner of items are thrown into it. Its job is simply to hold whatever is presented, which it does effortlessly, non-judgementally and without attachment.

The Chessboard Metaphor

The Chessboard Metaphor (described fully in Hayes et al., 1999) is another classic self-as-context metaphor in ACT. In this metaphor, the client is asked to imagine a chessboard that stretches out infinitely in all directions. On the chessboard sit pieces of two different colours, which are on opposing teams. The client is asked to consider if he sometimes feels like he is in a war between thoughts and feelings that often seem like they are on opposing sides of a contest or war. Within this metaphor, it is suggested that we often spend much of our time at the level of the pieces, trying to help the 'good' pieces triumph over the 'bad' pieces. However, the ACT therapist works with the client to identify that there is another perspective we may take – we can choose to participate at the level of the chessboard (as contrasted with the piece level), where we are in contact with all of the pieces, and all that is required is that we hold each of the pieces while we move forward in a direction that is consistent with our values. In the words of the band Green Day, the goal of this metaphor is to help the client learn how to become 'a conscientious objector to the war that's in my mind'. After introducing this metaphor, the therapist can then easily refer back to it by asking the client if she is currently at 'board level or piece level'.

Clouds in the Sky (Expanded)

It is also simple to follow the Clouds in the Sky mindfulness exercise described in the previous chapter with an addition to further illustrate the experience of self-as-context. For example, after a period of mindfulness with this exercise, the therapist can ask, 'And who is watching all of this unfold? Who is noticing the colour of the sky and the words on the clouds?' If the client is able to state something to the effect of, 'I am', then the therapist can clarify that this is the observing self-perspective. The therapist can also elaborate that even on days when the sky is especially cloudy, one may not be able to see the sky directly, but we all know that the sky is still there (Hayes et al., 1999). Within the parameters of this metaphor, the words written on the clouds are the conceptualized self or content, the process of simply observing the content and watching the clouds go by is ongoing self-awareness and the sky itself is the transcendent observing self. The fundamental nature of the sky is not affected by the clouds, and it is big enough to hold all of them, even when they are at their stormiest.

CONSIDERATIONS FOR WORKING WITH SELF-AS-CONTEXT

Because of its abstract nature, self-as-context work is not always simple for clients (or indeed for therapists!). Some clients are very concrete in their thinking and may never have considered existential or experiential questions about the nature of 'self'. For such clients, it may be confusing and not especially productive to spend much time on this component of ACT upfront. One approach with such clients would be to introduce the concept and experience with a few small exercises or metaphors, without being attached to achieving any particular clinical outcome. As long as the client can understand the basic concept of 'you are not your thoughts and feelings', the therapist can move on to other domains, looking for opportunities to reinforce the experience of self-as-context more organically throughout the later work of the therapy, referring back to the basic concepts as necessary.

On another note, some individuals with trauma histories may have significant difficulty with experiential exercises that focus on self-as-context. One common example can arise if the therapist chooses to do a closed eyes exercise to contact the observing self. As mentioned in the previous chapter on mindfulness, closed eyes exercises can be challenging for trauma survivors in general. However, this can especially be the case with self-as-context exercises, because they are explicitly designed to help the person disconnect or detach from his content and other private events. For those with a tendency toward severe avoidance, this type of exercise can quickly move from observing into dissociation. If the case conceptualization suggests that the client may be likely to have this type of reaction, then it is recommended that the therapist initially choose to focus on demonstrative metaphors that present the main points of self-as-context, without necessarily delving into long closed eyes exercises (good places to start are the 'House with Furniture in It' metaphor or the 'Progressive Self Questions' exercise). The therapist should also be prepared to quickly come back to grounding-type activities, such as the five senses mindfulness exercise described in the previous chapter, if the client begins to lose touch with a here-and-now focus.

Another way in which this work can be difficult for trauma survivors is if the individual grew up in an invalidating environment where he or she was not taught how to reliably label her own experiences (Kohlenberg and Tsai, 2007). If individuals have difficulty even labelling their experiences to be able to say 'I feel XYZ', then it can be extremely frustrating to ask them to tease their thoughts and feelings out as separate from a sense of self. For these individuals, preliminary work may first need to be done to assist them in being able to label their own experiences (Batten et al., 2005; Kohlenberg and Tsai, 2007). Ironically, it is these trauma survivors who may be most attached to or fused with their negative labels about themselves (e.g. 'I'm broken', 'I'm weak') and who may thus benefit the most from being able to recognize that they are not defined by their labels or history. For this reason, even though this may be especially challenging work for this group of clients, the therapist should not shy away from it simply because it can be difficult at times.

Although the work of identifying the self-as-context perspective may be initially challenging for both therapists and clients alike, it can be fundamentally transformative when individuals recognize experientially (not just verbally) that they are not defined by their thoughts, feelings and labels. This recognition can be experienced as truly expansive, as individuals come to find that they are 'big enough' to hold all of their experiences and that no emotion, thought or memory is so strong that it can destroy or harm them. The therapist will know that the client has truly caught on to this concept when the client is able to laugh at herself when she recognizes that she is operating from 'piece level' or uses the hand gesture of the yapping mouth (as described in Chapter 4) when she finds herself saying something that implies attachment to the conceptualized self.

Summary

One of the unique components of ACT is its focus on helping the individual find a different perspective from which to view thoughts, feelings, memories, urges and bodily sensations, rather than trying to change the content of those experiences directly. By contacting this observing self-as-context, it is hoped that individuals will come to recognize that they are not defined by their labels or private experiences and thus do not need to avoid or struggle with them. From the self-as-context perspective, the client is simply the container that holds all of the experiences as he or she moves forward in a valued direction.

Key Terms

Self-as-Content (otherwise known as the Conceptualized Self): a perspective from which the self is defined by one's self-evaluations, thoughts, feelings, memories and experiences.

Self-as-Context (otherwise known as the Observing Self): a perspective from which the self is experienced in a way that transcends the moment-to-moment content of one's private experiences.

Points for Review and Reflection

- How do you understand the difference between self-as-content and self-as-context?
- Do you think it would be more problematic to fuse with the positive or the negative aspects of one's conceptualized self? Give examples of how each could lead to problems.
- Which parts of your own conceptualized self would be most difficult for you to defuse from?

Further Reading

Harris, R. (2009) *ACT Made Simple*. Oakland, CA: New Harbinger Publications.

Hayes, S.C. (1984) Making sense of spirituality. *Behaviourism*, 12: 99–110.

Hayes, S.C., Strosahl, K.D. and Wilson, K.G. (1999) *Acceptance and Commitment Therapy: An Experiential Approach to Behaviour Change*. New York: Guilford Press.

Kohlenberg, R.J. and Tsai, M. (2007) *Functional Analytic Psychotherapy: Creating Intense and Curative Therapeutic Relationships*. New York: Springer.

Luoma, J.B., Hayes, S.C. and Walser, R.D. (2007) *Learning ACT: An Acceptance and Commitment Therapy Skills Training Manual for Therapists*. Oakland, CA: New Harbinger Publications.

7

Clarifying Individual Life Values

| Key Concepts |

- The primary work of ACT comes from individuals identifying those things in life – their chosen life values – that are most meaningful and important to them and then moving closer and closer to those values.
- This chapter provides a strong rationale for this focus on individual values and introduces multiple practical methods of helping clients to clarify and identify those things that are truly important to them.
- The difference between valued life directions and specific, achievable goals are highlighted, and techniques are provided that assist therapists and clients in distinguishing between the individual's chosen values and those promoted by the culture, parents or other significant individuals in the person's life.

Utilizing the perspectives and techniques described in the first half of this text, the primary work of ACT is focused on assisting clients to live their lives more effectively. This sounds simple enough, but how would one know whether or not someone's life were being effectively lived? Within the ACT model, each individual is able to mindfully choose the direction in which his life is headed, and the term 'values' is used to describe these chosen directions. It is through those individual values that one can determine workability. If specific choices or behaviours are functioning to move the individual closer to his values, then those choices are considered to be working effectively for the person. Conversely, if the things that a person is doing are taking him further and further from a life that he values, then his life is not currently seen as 'workable' as it is.

Because the word 'values' has been, at times, co-opted by different political and social action groups, it may sometimes be necessary to unpack these other connotations and defuse from them along with the client, in order to be able to use the term effectively in sessions. As the term is used in ACT, values are not about whether certain choices are right or wrong, or good or bad. Values are simply verbally construed descriptions of what is important to someone and where he or she wants to go in life (Hayes et al., 1999). Dahl et al. (2009: 9) further describe values as 'chosen concepts linked with patterns of action that provide a sense of meaning and that can coordinate our behaviour over long time frames'. From an ACT perspective, one's success in living is then defined by the extent to which our choices and behaviours are coordinated over time in a way that promotes the values we choose to see as important.

Values are considered to be relatively stable orientations that are chosen purposefully by the individual and are not determined by feelings that may change from moment to moment. One might have a wide range of feelings while behaving in accordance with one's values, and those feelings do not determine for the person whether the values that have been chosen are still valid. Similarly, values cannot be defined by fleeting thoughts or reactions about transient private events (e.g. 'I want to be at peace', 'I don't want to be anxious anymore'). Although values are not pursued as a way of contacting more pleasant thoughts, feelings and experiences, over time behaving in ways that are coherent with our values produces reinforcement that can make future similar behaviour more likely. That is, even when behaving in accordance with values doesn't feel good in the moment, our ability to use verbal behaviour can help us transform those experiences into ones that are considered more positive over time.

Everyone values something. Those who work clinically with ACT report that they have yet to find someone who has absolutely no values; however, some clients may have such a long history of avoidance or punishment by others for expressing their desires and preferences that they may have difficulty contacting their own values at first. The ACT core process described as values clarification is about working with the client to determine what he wants his life to move toward, rather than away from. For example, the ACT therapist would work with the substance abuser to stop moving away from the present moment or with the trauma survivor to stop orienting life in a way that avoids reminders of the traumatic event; instead, these individuals would be invited to shift their focus to what they would like to move toward in their lives now.

Within ACT, success is defined by living in accordance with our values, not by achieving specific goals (Harris, 2009). Although common language may not specifically distinguish between goals and values, ACT uses these terms to mean unique and distinct things. A value is seen as a general direction in which one wants to head in life, whereas a goal is a specific, achievable outcome that one can target in the service of a value. A common ACT metaphor that makes this distinction describes a value as a direction one might find on a compass, with the goals being specific stops along the way. For example, one could choose to make it important to move in the direction east. Moving continually in an eastward direction would be seen as a value, while moving from London to Berlin to Tokyo to San Francisco would be specific goals in the service of moving east. Regardless of how far east one travels, there is always more east that one can go. In the most basic sense, values are the compass directions that can guide our actions toward effective living.

Similarly, one might choose that being a reliable, compassionate friend is a core value. This might inform specific goals, such as attending a celebration for a friend, bringing a friend soup when she is sick and listening attentively when a friend describes a stressful situation she is experiencing. However, even once these specific goals have been accomplished, one can never say that 'being a good friend' is complete or has been achieved for all time. Values provide the directions and the bearing; goals are the specific, definable destinations along the way. A goal can be written down on a list of things to accomplish and eventually scratched off when the goal is achieved; a value can never be fully attained. More guidance for distinguishing between goals and values and targeting specific actions will be provided in Chapter 8.

IDENTIFYING CLIENT VALUES

In the most basic sense, values clarification practices are designed to help the client answer such questions as, 'What do you want your life to stand for? If you could have your life be about something – anything – what would it be?' For some clients, simply asking such a question directly will elicit the relevant information that the individual can share about her values and priorities. However, not everyone is introspective enough to be able to describe values immediately and simply in response to a direct question. For many individuals, metaphors and exercises can be especially helpful in identifying valued directions for living.

Stranded on a Desert Island/Memorial Service Exercise

This exercise capitalizes on the fact that nearing the end of life provides a natural time for self-reflection. Fortunately, because of the human capability for verbal behaviour, such reflection can happen at any point in one's actual lifespan, simply by bringing the idea to mind. There are many variants of such exercises in existential traditions and ACT. One such exercise (often done with eyes closed) can be initiated with directions such as the following:

'Imagine that you are on a long flight over a large body of water. Suddenly, half way through the flight, your plane is forced to make a crash landing onto a desert island. Everyone on the flight, including you, is able to survive the landing, but nobody back home knows that you are still alive, and it will be several weeks before you are eventually rescued. So, in the meantime, your family and friends go ahead and have a memorial service in your honour.

First, go ahead and imagine what the service would look like and who might be there. [Pause for a few moments.] Next, I'd like you to imagine that people begin to stand up to speak in your honour. However, rather than the universally positive things that might be more likely to be spoken at a memorial service, all of these people say what they would say based on how you have actually been living your life. They can magically see exactly what you've been valuing with your actions, and they speak the truth about that. I'll be quiet for a few minutes while you imagine what they might each say and then notice how it is for you to hear those things spoken by your loved ones. [The therapist is silent for 2–3 minutes.]

Next, I'd like you to imagine that you and the others have miraculously been rescued from the island, and you now have the chance to start over and begin your life again, based on your values, what's important to you and the insights you have gained from what you heard at the memorial service. Imagine moving through the next many years actually living with your actions as those that your values would suggest you do. [The therapist pauses for a few moments while the client pictures this.] Eventually, you die at a ripe old age, and your loved ones hold another memorial service for you. Listen now to what it is that your family and friends have to say and notice how it is to hear these things this time.'

The therapist pauses in silence for another 2–3 minutes and then processes the experience with the client.

Tombstone Exercise

A shorter version of the exercise above can be conducted by asking the client to imagine what would be written on his tombstone in the two sets of circumstances described above. It can be useful to actually provide two handouts with the outline of a tombstone on them and to ask the client to write different variants of what might describe the client's behaviour recently (e.g. 'Here lies Susan. She avoided as many uncomfortable situations as possible.') and in the circumstance where she has been living life in accordance with her values (e.g. 'Here lies Susan. She was always there for her friends and family when they needed her.'). The act of having to identify such discrepancies and write them plainly in black and white can be very powerful.

FORMAL VALUES CLARIFICATION EXERCISES

In addition to the imaginal values clarification exercises such as those described above, the ACT model also provides multiple opportunities for more formal values clarification work. For example, many clinicians will work with their clients using worksheets which list out multiple domains for values clarification. Several potential categories include:

- Intimate relationships
- Family relationships
- Social relationships
- Parenting
- Career/employment
- Education/personal growth
- Recreation and leisure
- Spirituality
- Citizenship/community
- Health and well-being
- Therapy.

This list is by no means all-inclusive or prescriptive. There is no rule that requires ACT therapists and clients to identify values in each of these areas. These are simply a grouping of valued domains that are frequently important to a wide variety of individuals. The therapist might suggest working on just a subset of these domains, or the therapist and client might choose to group certain domains together. For example, Dahl and colleagues (2009) describe a 'Bull's Eye' worksheet in which these areas are condensed into four valued domains: work and education, leisure, relationships, and personal growth and healing.

Regardless of the number of domains chosen for focus, the next step becomes to write out a brief narrative description of what the individual's values are in each domain. In this task, it is important to focus on what the client actually has control of in that area – his own behaviour! Thus, if the client is trying to describe values in different types of relationships, it is important to focus on how the client wishes to behave in the context of relationships – not on how he or she wants the other person in the relationship to behave. Similarly, when working on values in the context of employment, it is fine to identify the type of work the client wants (e.g. 'I want a job as a computer programmer'), but it is much more important to establish how he wishes to be as an employee and worker. Several examples of these types of values statements for a fictional client named Sophia are provided as models:

Parenting: I value being the type of parent who listens to my children, spends quality time with them, attends to their needs, demonstrates caring and love, and is accepting and non-critical.

Employment: I value being an employee who works hard to provide well for my family, seeks creative solutions, is innovative and who is an

<table>
<tr><td></td><td>effective leader, listening to my co-workers and challenging them to excel.</td></tr>
<tr><td>*Health*:</td><td>I value taking care of my physical self through regular exercise, being mindful of what I eat and getting sufficient sleep so that my body can rest and recover.</td></tr>
</table>

These are simply examples – the individual has the ability to determine which characteristics in which domains are the most important to him personally. Although this work is generally done in a verbal manner, it is important to point out that the words themselves are not of primary importance. The goal is not to focus on drafting the most eloquent values statements possible. In fact, it is not essential for the client to identify exactly the right words to convey his values, as long as the essence of the values is captured. With certain clients, the therapist will need to watch the process carefully to ensure that the client is not over-intellectualizing values to an extent that the heart of the process is being lost. For example, the highly verbal client may be overly focused on providing an inclusive list of adjectives and adverbs to describe a valued direction, either to achieve a 'perfect' values statement or to avoid strong emotions that may be triggered by the values clarification process.

When using the most traditional ACT values clarification worksheets, clients may be asked to provide quantitative measurements related to values in several ways. For example, each domain can be rated on overall importance (from 0 to 10), as well as the client's assessment of the extent to which he has been living his life with respect to each of those values over the past few months (from 0 to 10). After writing the values statements and rating them in this way, the therapist then has several courses to suggest where the next piece of work might be done most beneficially. For example, they could start by working on those valued domains that the client has rated as of highest importance, or with those domains where there is a high discrepancy between level of importance and level of consistency of behaviour with values.

There are multiple other methods for values assessment, many of which can be found free of charge at www.contextualpsychology.org. What is described above is the most traditional method that can be found in the original ACT text (Hayes et al., 1999). Therapists should feel free to experiment and try new ways of assessing values, depending on what might work best for a given clinical population. The format of such exercises or worksheets is not important; however, most values assessments should cover the main points described in this chapter.

CONSIDERATIONS IN VALUES CLARIFICATION

Ideally, values should be freely chosen, without avoidance, rigid rules or social manipulation (Luoma et al., 2007). However, as values clarification is an intrinsically verbal process, it is almost certain to initially call up content from the individual's history, including rules about how one 'should' or 'should not' behave. Thus, it is crucial for the therapist to intervene to prevent the client from simply identifying values based on what she believes will lead to approval by the client's parents, therapist or larger culture. This is a common initial issue that may come to light during values clarification work, due to a process known as pliance. In short, pliance is rule-governed behaviour in which an individual follows a rule, because she has been reinforced by others for following rules in the past (Dahl et al., 2009). It is natural for initial efforts at values clarification to be largely influenced by pliance. Thus, the therapist must be on the lookout for values statements that seem to be rote or inconsistent with other ideas that the client has previously expressed. If the therapist thinks that the client is stating values that are more about pliance with rules laid out by the culture, religious institutions or parents than about the client's deeper values, it can be very useful to ask questions such as, 'If nobody could ever know what you are writing here, what would you actually say?' or 'How much of what you've just identified is about you, and how much is about [the church, your parents, etc.]?' Pliance must also be carefully assessed for when determining specific goals that follow from the valued directions identified.

Over time, values may need to be prioritized and balanced. Even if all of the domains of valued living are evaluated as important by the client, it is not always possible to act in accordance with all of one's values at all times. Most certainly, there will be times when certain values that one has may come into conflict with one another. For example, the individual who values providing for her family through hard work may at times encounter values conflicts when the value of working hard means that she is not able to spend as much quality time with her family as she would choose in a world with no constraints. As has been stated in a biological example by Kelly Wilson (personal communication, 26 March 2010), both breathing and swallowing are very important to effective living. In some moments, breathing may be more important than swallowing, and in other moments swallowing may be more important than breathing. However, we are generally able to move back and forth flexibly between these two valued areas, recognizing that over time we can make them each important.

It is also possible that in some circumstances, the client's values may be significantly different from those held by the therapist. In general, this is not a tremendous problem. As described in Chapter 2, it is the stance of the ACT therapist to demonstrate radical respect for the client's values and the client's agency in identifying those values. In general, as long as the client's values do not involve harming self or others, most ACT therapists can work with most clients on attaining a life that is fulfilling based on the client's own values. The therapist should not be advocating for any particular agenda or expression of values. The focus in ACT is on workability, not on the therapist's own assumptions or beliefs. However, it is possible that, in certain cases, the therapist may hold fundamentally different things important, based on culture, religion or other traditions and experiences. It is the therapist's responsibility to be on the lookout for these sorts of potential conflicts and to seek consultation from other professionals about whether such differences can be appropriately worked through in the therapeutic context, or whether such a conflict may occasionally need to be resolved by assisting the client with finding another therapist.

An important note for the therapist concerns the potential sequencing of values work within different phases of ACT treatment. For example, some ACT practitioners choose to do values work at the beginning of therapy, while others choose to go through the work of willingness, mindfulness, self-as-context and defusion before attempting to germanely assist the client in identifying her values. There are currently no empirical data to guide this decision, and so such a determination should be made based on a careful case conceptualization for each client.

Many therapists may choose to briefly introduce the concept of values early in therapy and then come back to it in more detail later. Such an approach is based on the hypothesis that if individuals understand and can practise willingness and defusion, they may be more able to contact their own true values, rather than restating values that are based on rules or assumptions about what others would choose for them. On the other hand, if a client is reluctant to dive into work on the other processes in ACT, then it may help to say that the hard work that is being suggested is all designed to help the individual move forward with creating a life full of meaning, based on what is important to her specifically. The therapist may choose to return to the swamp metaphor that was described at the end of Chapter 3. Moving in the direction of one's values (the beautiful place on the other side of the swamp) is what makes going through something temporarily painful or unpleasant worthwhile and more than simply wallowing in the swamp. Furthermore, for some individuals who are court-ordered or otherwise mandated into treatment, they may not themselves identify that they have a problem to work on. Instead, they may respond more to a framework of identifying what is important to them and how they can use therapy to move their lives forward. For these individuals, beginning with values is often more productive than beginning with creative hopelessness and willingness.

Although building a valued life is a positive, constructive aspect of ACT, the work of values clarification can also be painful for some people. For example, if a client openly identifies how she truly wants to live her life, then she must also contact all of the times where she chose not to live in accordance with her values. The therapist should be watchful for this cascade of thinking and the resulting avoidance that can arise during values clarification. Similarly, if an individual believes that he could never really have the things that he values, then it can be very painful to acknowledge losses in the past or challenges in the future in these valued areas. For example, an individual who was a semi-professional athlete and has been permanently injured may feel that his values of physical fitness and participating in team sports are forever lost. It is important to begin by validating the tremendous losses he has experienced. However, over time, he and the therapist can work on exploring the underlying values of what was important to him as an athlete, and they can work on new ways to connect with those values in his current life. On the other hand, for many people, the work of values clarification can feel liberating and positive and can inspire individuals to recognize new ways that they can move forward with their lives immediately. In any of these cases, values clarification work done carefully can promote more connectedness between the therapist and client, which will serve the therapeutic dyad well for the work on committed action that will follow.

Summary

One of the unique aspects of ACT is its focus on working with the client to identify valued directions for her life. Moving toward one's values dignifies the hard work of willingness and committed action in the present moment. ACT therapists work with clients on values clarification using an array of metaphors, experiential practices and written exercises. The ACT approach is inherently respectful of individual differences and begins with the assumption that each individual has the right to determine what is important to her, as distinguished from the expectations of one's culture or authority figures.

Key Terms

Goals: specific, achievable outcomes that one can set forward to attain in the service of a valued direction for one's behaviour.

Pliance: rule-governed behaviour in which an individual follows a rule, because he has been reinforced by others for following rules in the past.

Values: verbally construed descriptions of what is important to someone and the direction he wants to go in specific domains of life.

Points for Review and Reflection

- How would you describe to a client the difference between a value and a goal? Why might it be useful to be able to look at things at both the level of a value and a goal?

(Continued)

(Continued)

- Provide two examples of clinical presentations that might be associated with clients having a hard time with the process of values clarification. How might these difficulties be addressed?
- What are your values as a therapist? How would you know whether you were moving toward your values in your work with clients?

Further Reading

Dahl, J.C., Plumb, J.C., Stewart, I. and Lundgren, T. (2009) *The Art and Science of Valuing in Psychotherapy: Helping Clients Discover, Explore, and Commit to Valued Action using Acceptance and Commitment Therapy.* Oakland, CA: New Harbinger Publications.

Hayes, S.C., Strosahl, K.D. and Wilson, K.G. (1999) *Acceptance and Commitment Therapy: An Experiential Approach to Behaviour Change.* New York: Guilford Press.

8

Building a Life through Committed Action

> ## Key Concepts
>
> - Once an individual's values are identified, the remainder of the work of ACT focuses on building larger and larger patterns of committed action that are consistent with those values.
> - The ACT therapist takes specific, practical steps to work with the client to identify appropriate behavioural targets for action, using the framework of 'Goals, Actions and Barriers'.
> - Specific guidelines are suggested for working with clients who may experience multiple barriers when working toward their chosen goals.

Despite the fact that many of the techniques described earlier in this book could be claimed by existential, humanistic, cognitive behavioural or even psychodynamic traditions, ACT is, at its core, a behavioural treatment. Thus, after clarifying the client's values, the majority of the work of ACT will focus on moving actively in the direction of those values by making, breaking and ultimately keeping commitments that lead to larger and larger patterns of committed actions in the service of those values. This work of moving forward on commitments requires the skills targeted in each of the other processes in ACT. For example, avoidance and fusion are frequent barriers to moving forward on commitments in valued directions, and thus defusion and willingness are essential skills to breaking through those barriers. Similarly, future-oriented commitments are best approached using present-moment awareness, with a consistent self-perspective that is not defined or challenged by thoughts, feelings and other reactions that are likely to arise as committed actions are targeted.

In fact, for many individuals, each step forward can be seen as its own type of exposure exercise. However, within ACT, the goal of exposure exercises is not seen as the reduction of anxiety or other reactions by repeated presentations of a specific stimulus. Instead, the goal of exposure is the same as the overall goal of ACT – to increase psychological flexibility. ACT-inspired exposure aims to broaden the individual's repertoire, so that he can move forward in a variety of ways that may be more functional in any given situation than avoidance or freezing would be. Thus, after an individual's values have been clarified and identified, commitment exercises (both in-session and as out-of-session homework) are the central focus of the rest of therapy. However, even if all domains of valued living were rated as highly important, one cannot begin working on everything all at once. Thus, the therapist and client can work together to choose two or three high priority areas and begin to identify goals there.

WORKING THROUGH GOALS, ACTIONS AND BARRIERS

Once the work of clarifying values in multiple domains has been accomplished, then the therapist and client can turn toward specific steps that can be taken to begin to bring the client's life more into alignment with those values. One framework for understanding how to take those next, concrete steps can be described as working on 'goals, actions and barriers'. As described in Chapter 7, goals are specific, achievable outcomes that one can set forward to attain in the service of a valued direction for one's life. Actions are then the smaller steps that one would have to take in order to accomplish those goals. Finally, as one works toward taking actions and achieving specific goals, it is inevitable that barriers will be presented that make the accomplishment of those actions challenging. The process described below will lay out practical strategies for working through both internal and external barriers to effective action.

As a practical example, let's say that a 35-year-old mother of two, Sophia, has completed a full values assessment, as laid out in Chapter 7. In addition to identifying her values in 10 domains, she has also rated each of those domains in terms of importance, and with respect to how consistently she has lived her life in accordance with those values over the past three months. Upon reviewing her values clarification worksheets, the therapist suggests to Sophia that they begin by targeting three areas in which to begin identifying specific goals: Parenting and Employment because they both have very high ratings on importance, and Health and Well-being because this area has the largest discrepancy between importance and the level of consistency with that value in the last three months. Sophia's values were used as an example in Chapter 7 and are described again here, along with her ratings for each of the three domains:

Parenting:	I value being the type of parent who listens to my children, spends quality time with them, attends to their needs, demonstrates caring and love, and is accepting and non-critical. Importance: 10; Consistency: 6.
Employment:	I value being an employee who works hard to provide well for my family, seeks creative solutions, is innovative and who is an effective leader, listening to my co-workers and challenging them to excel. Importance: 9; Consistency: 6.
Health and well-being:	I value taking care of my physical self through regular exercise, being mindful of what I eat and getting sufficient sleep so that my body can rest and recover. Importance: 8; Consistency: 2.

Once the set of values that will be addressed first has been identified, the next step is to begin to specify goals and actions that the individual can take in order to move forward in those areas. Luoma et al. (2007) identify several characteristics of goals that are likely to be workable: (1) they should be specific and measurable; (2) they should be practical and within the client's ability to accomplish; (3) they should involve something more than what a dead man could do (Lindsley, 1968); (4) they should be committed to publicly (at least in the presence of the therapist); (5) they should be on target with the values of the client; and (6) they should be linked to the functional needs of the client. These goals can be of any magnitude – even tiny goals are meaningful, as long as they are in the direction of the individual's values. Small, successive approximations can be seen as planting the seeds of committed action. The fruits of these actions may not be immediately visible, but as with a real garden, the pay-off for hard work in committing and tending to the small seeds is only apparent over time. The most important factor is to build effective patterns of action over time that are consistent with one's values.

Within each of those goals, there are specific actions that follow that would need to be taken in order for the goal to be achieved. In the case of Sophia, a sample of her goals and specific actions to facilitate those goals are as follows (Note that only one goal per value is provided here for brevity but, in reality, each valued domain could have several goals and actions.):

Parenting

Goal 1 – I will regularly spend time reading with my children (at least four times per week).
Action 1 – I will leave work by 5:30 p.m. each day.
Action 2 – I will set limits and turn off the television by 7:30 p.m. each day.

Employment

Goal 1 – I will take on two new challenges at work each month to face with creativity and innovation.
Action 1 – I will speak up in staff meetings at least once per week, rather than hiding from my boss's attention.

Action 2 – when given a task I'm not sure how to tackle, I will explore the issue and do research rather than trying to pass the task on to someone else.

Health and well-being

Goal 1 – I will be mindful of what I eat during the day, rather than mindlessly eating when I feel stressed or bored.
Action 1 – I will bring healthy snacks from home to eat throughout the day.
Action 2 – when I feel stressed at work, I will practise mindfulness for five minutes, rather than immediately turning to food for comfort.

After goals and actions have been identified, the final step in planning is to try to predict and undermine the likely barriers that could potentially get in the way of following through with the identified actions. These barriers are generally the same types of things that have gotten in the way of actions in the past, and thus clients are generally experts in recognizing those potential barriers. Such barriers can be categorized in a practical manner as being either external or internal. If the barrier is external, then this leads to the identification of additional actions that can be taken to contribute to the success of the commitment, whereas if the barrier is internal (responses to thoughts, feelings or urges), then this points to the need to revisit willingness, defusion and mindfulness skills.

For example, with Sophia's goal to eat in a more healthy and mindful way throughout the day, she was able to identify several potential barriers to following through with the identified actions. First, she identified that she didn't always have healthy food on hand at home, and that she was frequently running late in the morning without time to pack food to take with her to work. These were both classified as external barriers to action, and two additional actions were added to this goal: going to the grocery store each weekend to stock up on healthy snacks, and setting her alarm clock 10 minutes earlier to have time to pack food for the day. In addition, she identified some internal barriers that could subvert her actions, including the recognition that during the afternoon, she was prone to giving in to thoughts such as, 'I have so little energy right now. I just need a little sugar to pick me up'. Her therapist worked with her to identify several defusion exercises she could easily practise at her desk when those sorts of thoughts arose. They also identified that unwillingness to experience frustration and anxiety are frequent internal barriers for Sophia during the week, and thus the therapist reintroduced the importance of practising willingness to experience the full range of emotions and sensations in the service of Sophia's values.

Although clients are generally aware of their routine barriers, there are sometimes barriers that are not as easily identified. If there seems to be an unidentified barrier, over and over, to following through with a specific commitment, then it might require taking this barrier apart again to ensure that there is not some sort of ambivalence – that the client is not choosing this goal for reasons of pliance or to follow a perceived expectation, rather than because it is what he truly values. Take the example of the young male client who said for months that he wanted to go back to school and earn an advanced degree. The initial action chosen was going to obtain a course prospectus from a local college. However, the client returned to the session week after week without meeting that action. When the therapist revisited this goal with him in more detail after weeks of not meeting his commitment, he was eventually able to share that he had romantic feelings for the therapist and thought that she would only like a man with a college degree. After working through this issue in a new way, he expressed that he might eventually like to go back to school, but it really wasn't important to him right now.

Pausing in the Moment

Experiential exercises can also be used to identify barriers to committed action. For example, individuals can be asked to close their eyes and identify a committed action they have been struggling with and trying to work on. For example, Sophia could be asked to focus on that moment, mid-afternoon, where she has a choice about whether to momentarily self-soothe by eating junk food or to slow down, practise mindfulness and then choose to eat something healthy if she truly is hungry. In her imagination, Sophia would be asked to spend two or three minutes simply pausing in that moment just before she makes her choice, in order to watch with curiosity the thoughts, feelings and other sensations that arise. Then, she could imagine making the choice that is not consistent with her values and watching what reactions come forward. Next, she could be asked to rewind the image back to the choice point and picture herself choosing the values-consistent option, again watching what thoughts, feelings and reactions are present. Going inside these experiences and watching the responses non-judgementally creates yet another way to assist with determining the barriers and possible reinforcers of acting in a values-consistent manner.

The process of addressing internal barriers also provides a useful opportunity to return to the exercise of writing down thoughts on cards, reinforcing the lessons described in Chapters 3 and 4. If the client can identify several potential internal barriers that could get in the way of following through with committed action, then she can again practise writing down those thoughts, feelings and urges on paper and reminding herself that she can relate to them in multiple different ways. When those thoughts and feelings arise, she does not have to automatically give in to them. Instead, she can hold them and carry them around without having to fight them or believe them. It can be useful to first do this again in the session as it relates to specific committed actions, writing down any potential private events that could become challenging in the moment, giving the client the opportunity to practise seeing these reactions as content that she carries around with her, rather than as overwhelming thoughts and feelings that she has to give in to.

CONSIDERATIONS IN WORKING ON COMMITTED ACTION

In support of the model described in this chapter, it can be very helpful to have basic worksheets for the client to use to organize goals, actions and barriers in an easy-to-follow format. Examples can be found in Hayes et al. (1999) or on www.contextualpsychology.org. However, it is not required that any specific worksheet or written format must be used when working on commitments. At the same time, it can at least be useful to write down what the person commits to doing each week, providing a copy for both client and therapist at the end of each session. This level of public commitment can assist with follow-through in action. However, the therapist must also ensure that he follows up to ask about the status of the committed actions in the following session. It can be very demoralizing when the therapist forgets or doesn't bother to ask about whether the client has followed through with the commitment from the past week. ACT therapists obviously work to reduce pliance, even to perceived rules provided by the therapist, but by assisting the client with follow-up, therapists can help model effective ways to monitor behaviour and be accountable to oneself. Similarly, if doing this work in group therapy, it can be useful to have each group member (including the therapist) make public commitments and then follow up the next week. Within such a structure, the other members of the group need to also be prepared not to rescue, judge or overly praise the individual based on whether he does or does not follow through with the commitment the following week.

The issue of how the therapist can work to respond non-judgementally, regardless of whether or not the client follows through on a given commitment, will be addressed in more detail in Chapter 11. However, it is important to clarify the general approach that the ACT therapist takes toward client commitments. The therapist works to clarify that when one makes a commitment, it is not a promise or a prediction that one can make with certainty, but a general stance that is in alignment with contributing to a valued life. Even if someone is 100 per cent committed in the moment that the commitment is made, we all fall short sometimes. It may be useful to return to the metaphor of learning to ride a bicycle referenced earlier in this text. Riding a bicycle requires balance and relies upon the general value of remaining upright, but it is not an all-or-nothing action in which one will always be fully upright. Sometimes the rider will be off balance to one side, sometimes to the other side. However, it is extremely important that cyclists be committed to remaining upright as a general direction, even though they will hover slightly off from vertical at multiple times during each ride. Furthermore, if the rider falls, there is another choice point. He can choose to lie on the ground, analysing exactly how he got there, or complaining about the unfairness of the bumps in the road. Or, as with committed action in ACT, he can choose to recognize where he is now and get back up to keep moving in the valued direction. The results of any particular action are never certain; thus, ACT requires a commitment to the process of valued living and mindful action, not to an unpredictable outcome. In sum, committed action requires a willingness to take risks, when those risks occur in the service of living in a way that is consistent with one's values.

Furthermore, although commitments are specific and about moving toward a particular goal, they have to be flexible enough to incorporate new information or changes in circumstances without judgement. It may not always appear that one is making progress. Returning to the metaphor of riding a bicycle up a mountain from Chapter 2, if one is riding up a particularly difficult or uncharted path, one may sometimes need to move back down part of the mountain to find another path, rather than doggedly continuing up a path that is treacherous or impassable. The client must learn to have faith that sometimes even moving down the mountain in the short term can be in the service of moving effectively up the mountain in the long term. The effectiveness of any action is not measured solely in one moment. Instead, the client must ask herself on an ongoing basis: if I take this next action, is it in the service of bringing me closer to or further from my chosen values in the long term?

Overall, for commitments to change to be successful, individuals must be willing to accept responsibility for changing their own lives. For some clients, this may mean that they need to recognize any investment they may have in keeping things the way they are. It may seem counter-intuitive that someone would stay stuck or continue to live in ways that are not working if she had other options. However, for some people who have truly been 'wronged' by someone else, it can feel like they will let the other individual who has wronged them 'off the hook' if they are able to move forward. Most people are not cognizant of the fact that they may be holding on to 'reasons' such as this for not taking action to move their lives forward. However, through defusion and metaphor, the skilful ACT therapist can carefully point out these somewhat perverse contingencies for staying stuck without invalidating the client's truly real and valid pain.

Although the focus on committed action will seem altogether practical and straightforward to some therapists, other therapists who are new to behavioural ways of conducting therapy may not feel comfortable with such a directive style in therapy. Some clinicians do not initially gravitate to the commitment component of ACT, because they themselves are not as willing to work with clients to pin down specific goals each session. This is another example of how it is important for therapists to watch their own reactions in the session and ensure that they themselves are not shying away from certain pieces of work that bring up personal feelings of discomfort. ACT therapists are reminded that working with the client to identify very specific goals and actions is in the service of the client's self-defined values, and if the client's characteristic ways of approaching such circumstances were going to work, they would have done so already. Even very straightforward and directive portions of ACT are in the service of the client's best interests.

Summary

Beyond the metaphors, exercises and tools of ACT, the core of this behavioural therapy involves assisting the client with moving forward with his life in valued ways. The ACT therapist works with each client to identify specific goals that are important destinations along the client's valued directions. Each goal can be further broken down into clearly defined actions that clients can take to move forward. The ACT model then assists clients with developing plans to address both internal and external barriers to progress along those dimensions, creating larger and larger patterns of committed action over time.

Key Terms

Actions: smaller, practical steps that one takes in order to accomplish one's larger goals.

Barriers: internal or external challenges that could get in the way of accomplishing valued actions if not effectively addressed.

Points for Review and Reflection

- Describe how you would respond to a client who asked you, 'Why should I even bother committing to do these things? I always fail at everything I set out to do'.
- What are two different ways that the therapist could work with a client on identifying potential barriers to effective action?
- How would you distinguish between an internal and external barrier? Depending on that analysis, how would you then approach internal and external barriers differently with a client?

Further Reading

Dahl, J.C., Plumb, J.C., Stewart, I. and Lundgren, T. (2009) *The Art and Science of Valuing in Psychotherapy: Helping Clients Discover, Explore, and Commit to Valued Action Using Acceptance and Commitment Therapy*. Oakland, CA: New Harbinger Publications.

Hayes, S.C., Strosahl, K.D. and Wilson, K.G. (1999) *Acceptance and Commitment Therapy: An Experiential Approach to Behaviour Change*. New York: Guilford Press.

9

ACT for Anxiety

Key Concepts

- Working with anxiety disorders provides one of the most straightforward opportunities to practise ACT and all of its processes.
- Anxiety has a distinctly future-oriented, verbal component at its core, which makes the ACT approach a particularly relevant model for the treatment of anxiety disorders, including panic disorder, obsessive compulsive disorder (OCD) and post-traumatic stress disorder.
- As with all effective treatments for anxiety disorders, ACT incorporates exposure exercises, but with a focus on increasing psychological flexibility and valued living, rather than decreasing anxiety.

Since the inception of ACT in its original form as 'Comprehensive Distancing' in the early 1980s, anxiety disorders have been seen as a highly appropriate clinical target for ACT. One important reason for a focus on anxiety disorders is simply because of their high prevalence in the general population (Narrow et al., 2002) and high rates of chronicity and associated functional impairment. In addition, although there are several existing effective treatments for anxiety disorders (see Barlow [2002] for detailed descriptions of these primarily cognitive behavioural approaches), a significant number of individuals who receive traditional treatments fail to respond, and even responders often report notable symptoms and problems in functioning after treatment (Orsillo et al., 2004). Importantly, there are several aspects of an ACT-based model that are extremely relevant to the conceptualization of anxiety disorders (Eifert and Forsyth, 2005; Forsyth and Eifert, 2007); this chapter will focus on those aspects of the application of ACT to anxiety disorders that are most notable.

USING ACT WITH ANXIETY DISORDERS

To begin with, the conceptualization of what may cause and maintain anxiety disorders is very consistent with an ACT model, in that anxiety disorders have unwillingness and avoidance at their very core. Individuals with anxiety disorders may take heroic steps to avoid internal bodily sensations associated with panic, feelings such as fear and anxiety, and all manner of situations and circumstances that are likely to occasion anxiety and its correlates. Thus, a model of psychopathology that has experiential avoidance at its core is extremely relevant for this category of problems. It is certainly natural up to a certain point to try to avoid experiences that raise anxiety and fear; however, when strategies of avoidance and escape begin to be applied rigidly and inflexibly to anxiety and fear, as well as to the situations that are likely to trigger such reactions, then normal anxiety and fear may begin to become 'disordered' (Eifert and Forsyth, 2005). Barlow's (2002) well-known model of anxious apprehension can easily be viewed through an ACT lens. In this model, anxiety is described as 'a future-oriented mood state in which one is ready or prepared to attempt to cope with upcoming negative events' (Barlow, 2002: 64). This model goes on to describe two primary methods of attempting to cope with anxiety: (1) avoidance of situations that provoke anxiety or the internal experiences of anxiety; and (2) heightened attempts at planning and problem solving through worry in an attempt to avoid negative affect. Based on this analysis, the dual concentration in ACT on reducing avoidance and decreasing fusion with cognitive content is especially germane.

For the anxious client who presents with a focus on avoiding anxiety at all costs, the application of ACT is generally marked by a strong emphasis in the early stages on the creative hopelessness and willingness aspects of treatment. Such clients have been treating their anxiety as if it is something very dangerous. Thus, the therapist will work carefully to demonstrate the futility of struggling with anxiety. The quicksand metaphor and other exercises identified in Chapter 3 are core interventions for this purpose. Clients who have been struggling with anxiety for long periods of time have generally tried many different things in order to avoid or escape their anxiety, resorting to a wide variety of efforts at internal and external control. It can be helpful for the therapist to ask a question such as, 'When you consider just how much time, effort and energy you have put into trying to get rid of anxiety, doesn't it seem a little strange that it hasn't gotten any better – that, in fact, it may have even gotten worse? With any other project or goal in life, if you had put this much effort in, don't you think you would have seen results by now?' Clients may not know what to make of this line of questioning at first, but they are generally able to relate to the experience described, in which the harder they have tried to rid themselves of anxiety, the worse the anxiety has become.

This work of Creative Hopelessness is truly key for working with anxiety disorders, as individuals with these problems have been trying desperately over time to do anything they can not to experience anxiety and other related thoughts, feelings and bodily sensations. It can thus seem terrifying when the therapist (whether in ACT or in CBT) asks the client to begin to approach those experiences that the client has made extraordinary efforts to avoid at all costs. Through metaphors and exercises, the ACT therapist seeks to help clients recognize that control efforts have not truly been working to reduce their anxiety over time anyway and may have even made things more problematic.

Another feature of anxiety disorders that makes an ACT approach particularly relevant is the fact that anxiety and worry are typically very future-focused. By definition, the future can only be imagined because of the verbal abilities that allow humans to project forward in time in their imagination. Because of this excessive fixation on the future, approaches that are focused on mindfulness and present-moment awareness are very appropriate for ACT treatment of anxiety disorders. CBT approaches also recognize the role of thoughts and other verbal behaviour in the spectrum of anxiety disorders. However, rather than asking clients to explore the accuracy of and evidence for their thoughts, ACT practitioners work with their clients to begin to defuse from these thoughts and see them for what they are (e.g. 'milk, milk, milk, milk'). Thoughts such as, 'my heart is beating so fast that I might die', are not examined for the probability that the content of the thought will actually come true. Instead, the ACT therapist uses defusion exercises to demonstrate that minds are simply thought-generating machines, and we do not have to take their products literally.

Once these concepts have been introduced, then ACT-based approaches to anxiety will feature a strong focus on the most reliably effective component of existing approaches to the treatment of anxiety: exposure. As described in Chapter 8, ACT-based exposure efforts are not targeted toward habituation or the extinction of anxiety responses. Instead, the rationale of increasing psychological and behavioural flexibility is provided. Such exposure work can be done in vivo, imaginally or interoceptively with the client's own bodily sensations. Regardless of the type of exposure practised, the ACT therapist will suggest that if it is the case that avoidance and struggle have gotten the individual more and more stuck, then the antidote to this problem is finding a new way to approach these experiences.

Interoceptive exposure is used in many common approaches to anxiety disorder treatment. In such practices, the client is instructed to engage in a variety of low-risk physical activities (e.g. spinning in a chair, breathing through a straw, hyperventilating) that are likely to produce the internal experiences of anxiety and panic. An ACT approach might use several of these very same techniques to bring about the private experiences associated with anxiety, either in the session or as homework.

However, rather than teaching the client ways of reducing anxiety when these symptoms are present and suggesting that anxiety symptoms will go down over time with practice, the ACT therapist will use these opportunities to coach the client on practising willingness and acceptance, rather than avoidance and escape. Glaser and colleagues (2009) suggest that the breath-holding exercise from *Get Out of Your Mind and Into Your Life* (Hayes and Smith, 2005) can be used in this way as well. For example, the client may be asked to attempt to hold his breath for as long as he can, without providing any additional instructions, assuming that the client will naturally begin by using his characteristic avoidance and control strategies. Later in the same session or later in a course of treatment, the client can again be asked to practise holding his breath, but from a stance of acceptance, in which he chooses to be willing to experience the sensations and feelings that arise without fusing with his catastrophic thoughts. In addition to seeing which method leads the client to be able to hold his breath longer, he is also encouraged to share what was different about those two approaches to experiencing challenging thoughts, feelings and bodily sensations.

Although willingness and defusion are essential components of an ACT-based treatment for anxiety disorders, it is important to remember the role of values in motivating the hard work of exposure and acceptance. As described above, it can be terrifying to ask individuals who have been fighting anxiety to begin to face and approach their 'anxiety monsters'. On the part of the therapist, it would not be fair to ask the client to do so without a valid means of justifying such hard work. In ACT, the motivating factor is the idea that by letting go of avoidance and control, the client has the possibility of regaining a life that she can truly value. The idea of being able to move forward with flexibility in the service of those things that are important to the client is what makes the hard work of exposure worthwhile. However, this concept may initially be difficult for some clients, because their chronic avoidance may have led to significant levels of value constriction. Because these clients have spent so long revolving their lives around their unwillingness to experience anxiety, it may initially be challenging to have clients identify what is truly important to them. However, when individuals realize that there is a possibility that they can regain their lives, it can be exceptionally powerful. For this reason, Orsillo and colleagues (2004) suggest that the idea of values-based action be introduced early in therapy and reinforced throughout the course of treatment when working with individuals with anxiety problems.

EMPIRICAL SUPPORT FOR ACT WITH ANXIETY (SELECTED READINGS)

Batten, S.V. and Hayes, S.C. (2005) Acceptance and Commitment Therapy in the treatment of comorbid substance abuse and post-traumatic stress disorder: a case study. *Clinical Case Studies*, 4: 246–62.

Block, J.A. and Wulfert, E. (2000) Acceptance or change: treating socially anxious college students with ACT or CBGT. *The Behaviour Analyst Today*, 1: 1–55.

Carrascoso López, F.J. (2000) Acceptance and Commitment Therapy (ACT) in panic disorder with agoraphobia: a case study. *Psychology in Spain*, 4: 120–8.

Dalrymple, K.L. and Herbert, J.D. (2007) Acceptance and Commitment Therapy for generalized social anxiety disorder: a pilot study. *Behaviour Modification*, 31: 543–68.

Eifert, G.H., Forsyth, J.P., Arch, J., Espejo, E., Keller, M. and Langer, D. (2009) Acceptance and Commitment Therapy for anxiety disorders: three case studies exemplifying a unified treatment protocol. *Cognitive and Behavioural Practice*, 16: 368–85.

Roemer, L., Orsillo, S.M. and Salters-Pedneault, K. (2008) Efficacy of an acceptance-based behaviour therapy for generalized anxiety disorder: evaluation in a randomized controlled trial. *Journal of Consulting and Clinical Psychology*, 76: 1083–9.

Twohig, M.P. (2009a) Acceptance and Commitment Therapy for treatment-resistant posttraumatic stress disorder: a case study. *Cognitive and Behavioural Practice*, 16: 243–52.

Twohig, M.P. (2009b) The application of Acceptance and Commitment Therapy to obsessive-compulsive disorder. *Cognitive and Behavioural Practice*, 16: 18–28.

Twohig, M.P., Hayes, S.C. and Masuda, A. (2006) Increasing willingness to experience obsessions: Acceptance and Commitment Therapy as a treatment for obsessive-compulsive disorder. *Behaviour Therapy*, 37: 3–13.

Williams, L.M. (2007) Acceptance and Commitment Therapy: an example of third-wave therapy as a treatment for Australian Vietnam War veterans with posttraumatic stress disorder (PTSD). *Salute*, 19: 13–15.

ACT FOR PANIC DISORDER AND AGORAPHOBIA

When treating individuals who meet the criteria for panic disorder, with or without agoraphobia, there are several ACT-specific targets. First, individuals with panic disorder evaluate their somatic symptoms as very dangerous and thus practise multiple methods of experiential and behavioural avoidance to go out of their way not to experience panic-like sensations. They also worry excessively about the potential for future panic attacks and the negative consequences of the attacks. Furthermore, when agoraphobia is also present, the individual's life becomes so constricted that behaviour is constrained within smaller and smaller limits in order to avoid any situation that is perceived as potentially unsafe and in which he might experience a panic attack.

Thus, the ACT approach to treating panic disorder is very straightforward, incorporating all of the six core ACT processes. Acceptance and willingness techniques from the perspective of self-as-context are presented as the alternative to the avoidance strategies that have led to the client's increasingly constrained life. Defusion strategies are used to assist the client in finding a new way to respond to excessive worry thoughts about the likelihood and consequences of future panic attacks. Finally, much of the work of therapy then revolves around exposure efforts designed to help expand the client's life in valued directions, so that the client can increase valued living and committed action, rather than remaining stuck due to an almost exclusive use of avoidance and escape strategies. It is important to note that these exposure exercises can be limited by time or by situation, but not by level of distress. That is, the individual could choose to practise willingness for five seconds or five minutes, or to begin by practising willingness in a specific circumstance or location. However, it should not be the case that the exposure exercise is allowed to end simply because the individual is feeling highly anxious or uncomfortable. Perpetuating escape from anxiety in this way simply reinforces the client's perception that there is a level of anxiety that he is not able to experience and cements the avoidance agenda even further.

ACT FOR OBSESSIVE COMPULSIVE DISORDER

Another anxiety disorder that can be seen productively through an ACT conceptualization is obsessive compulsive disorder, as both the obsessions and related compulsions suggest specific ACT targets. First, individuals who meet the criteria for OCD experience more than just average worry thoughts; instead they report thoughts that are extremely intrusive, unreasonable and at times bizarre. Such thoughts are experienced by the individual as highly distressing and lead to significant attempts to avoid or escape the cognitions. In ACT terminology, these individuals are highly fused with their obsessive thoughts. The associated compulsions in this disorder are then seen as repeated behaviours that are engaged in to reduce the frequency of, or distress related to, the individual's obsessions. As with the treatment of all anxiety disorders, the ACT approach to OCD involves working with the client to experience the obsessive thoughts as just thoughts, the anxiety as a feeling that the client can be safely willing to experience, and then using these strategies as the individual focuses on moving forward with his life, rather than engaging in compulsions designed to eliminate obsessive thoughts or anxious feelings (Twohig, 2009b; Twohig et al., 2006). Many of the methods of exposure and response prevention (Foa and Franklin, 2001) can be utilized in ACT treatment for OCD; however, as with all ACT-infused exposure, the focus is on developing a broad and flexible repertoire of behaviour in the presence of the feared experience, rather than on the habituation of anxious responding.

ACT FOR POST-TRAUMATIC STRESS DISORDER

PTSD is the only anxiety disorder that is seen as having a specific precipitating event. Following a given traumatic event, the individual who meets criteria for PTSD develops multiple symptoms in clusters that can be categorized as intrusive experiences, avoidance/numbing symptoms and hyperarousal. The original conceptualization of PTSD as an anxiety disorder has led to several effective treatments that generally incorporate an exposure component. However, it has also been argued from an acceptance-based perspective that PTSD can be more usefully conceptualized as a disorder of experiential avoidance (Batten et al., 2005; Orsillo and Batten, 2005). From this more recent perspective, PTSD symptoms are viewed within a model that suggests that chronic, broad-based efforts to avoid thoughts, feelings and memories related to the traumatic event produce a long-term escalation of these private events and related functional impairments.

ACT-based interventions for PTSD (Follette and Pistorello, 2007; Walser and Westrup, 2007) apply the general ACT approach described throughout this text, with several specific nuances. For example, as described in earlier chapters, individuals with childhood trauma histories may have problems with identifying a sense of self or may not be able to label and identify their feelings or personal values early in treatment. This may happen either because these clients were never shaped to have those skills in their repertoire or because they were actively punished for expressing needs and wants, and the ACT therapist can work with these clients to bolster the repertoire of labelling self-experiences. Additionally, the ACT model is proposed to have particular relevance and flexibility for the treatment of post-traumatic problems in living, because it can make use of exposure exercises and willingness practices with respect to traumatic memories and reminders, but it can also focus much more on the present and on living a life of meaning (rather than focusing on the traumatic past) than many other approaches (Batten et al., 2005; Walser and Westrup, 2007).

ACT WITH OTHER ANXIETY DISORDERS

Although applications of ACT for Panic Disorder, OCD and PTSD have been specifically highlighted above, an ACT-informed approach can also have significant relevance for other anxiety disorders as well. For example, Orsillo and Roemer have developed a coherent acceptance- and mindfulness-based approach to the treatment of generalized anxiety disorder (GAD), and they have published multiple empirical and theoretical descriptions of this treatment (Orsillo and Roemer, in press; Roemer and Orsillo, 2005; Roemer et al., 2008). Promising preliminary results have also been found to support an ACT-based conceptualization and treatment for social anxiety disorder and related problems (Block and Wulfert, 2000; Dalrymple and Herbert, 2007). Because of the strong theoretical framework based on experiential avoidance, cognitive fusion and values constriction that can be applied to all anxiety disorders, ACT may be particularly relevant to this class of problems in functioning.

CONSIDERATIONS FOR USING ACT WITH ANXIETY DISORDERS

One barrier to progress in any treatment for anxiety disorders is the underlying level of generalized avoidance in which clients engage. In addition to its role in developing and maintaining the anxiety problems that have brought the individual to treatment, a high level of avoidance can also interfere with engagement in treatment, by leading to clients avoiding practising homework exercises or even to a pattern of missed therapy appointments, because the therapy itself is perceived as being associated with anxiety and thus aversive. In ACT, these issues with avoidance of therapy or therapeutic exercises and homework are not seen as problems. Instead, they are seen as an excellent opportunity to examine the very specific barriers that are interfering with the client's life. By engaging with these barriers openly and non-judgementally, therapist and client can work together to identify important patterns of the client's behaviour that keep her stuck in her life as it is.

As with many problems that are addressed in ACT treatment, anxiety disorders can be productively addressed in either individual or group therapy (e.g. Batten et al., 2009; Glaser et al., 2009). Although an individual therapy approach may allow for personalized and in-depth exploration of the client's values and barriers, group therapy for anxiety disorders can also be particularly useful in helping to defuse and normalize thoughts that symptoms of anxiety are unusual or dangerous in some way. In addition, group-based treatment can allow for the learning of ACT principles through other individuals' experiences. Further, the social context of group therapy naturally provides opportunities for in vivo exposure to social anxiety, which may promote the subsequent willingness to experience anxiety in an interpersonal setting.

One final consideration related to ACT-based treatment of anxiety disorders relates to the therapeutic stance of the treatment provider in ACT. Consistent with the model of therapist behaviour outlined in Chapter 3, an ACT approach to treating problems related to anxiety provides a unique opportunity for the therapist to provide novel responses to anxiety and related cognitions. For example, an ACT therapist might respond irreverently ('Wow, that's a brilliant example of fusion!') to a client's report that he almost vomited during an anxiety-provoking situation in the past week. Such unexpected responses to content that would generally be seen as negative can model for the client the core message of ACT: 'Your thoughts, feelings and bodily sensations are not the enemy – it is the struggle against them that keeps you stuck'.

Summary

Although many effective treatments for anxiety disorders currently exist, none is universally effective; ACT is proposed as one model that may address several of the gaps in extant treatments. Across diagnostic criteria, the ACT model of treatment is generally consistent for each of the anxiety disorders: individuals are shown that private experiences and bodily sensations can be approached with willingness, rather than avoidance; defusion methods are used to change the characteristic response to troubling thoughts; and exposure practices in and out of session assist the individual with moving forward with a valued life, whether or not anxiety is present.

Key Term

Exposure exercises: in ACT, exposure exercises can be any opportunity for an individual to practise approaching a situation or sensation that she characteristically attempts to avoid, control or escape, instead practising willingness and defusion in the service of broadening her behavioural repertoire in the presence of the avoided stimulus.

Points for Review and Reflection

- What is the difference in the way that exposure exercises are practised in ACT versus traditional CBT?
- Why is a focus on values so important when implementing ACT for the treatment of anxiety disorders?
- Provide at least two theoretical reasons why ACT would be a potentially appropriate and effective treatment for anxiety disorders.

Further Reading

Eifert, G.H. and Forsyth, J.P. (2005) *Acceptance and Commitment Therapy for Anxiety Disorders: A Practitioner's Treatment Guide to Using Mindfulness, Acceptance, and Values-based Behaviour Change Strategies*. Oakland, CA: New Harbinger Publications.

Forsyth, J.P. and Eifert, G.H. (2007) *The Mindfulness and Acceptance Workbook for Anxiety: A Guide to Breaking Free from Anxiety, Phobias and Worry using Acceptance and Commitment Therapy*. Oakland, CA: New Harbinger Publications.

Glaser, N.M., Blackledge, J.T., Shepherd, L.M. and Dean, F.P. (2009) Brief group ACT for anxiety. In J. Blackledge, J. Ciarrochi and F. Dean (eds), *Acceptance and Commitment Therapy: Current Directions* (pp. 175–200). Queensland, Australia: Australian Academic Press.

Orsillo, S.M., Roemer, L., Block-Lerner, J., LeJeune, C. and Herbert, J.D. (2004) ACT with anxiety disorders. In S.C. Hayes and K.D. Strosahl (eds), *A Practical Guide to Acceptance and Commitment Therapy* (pp. 103–32). New York: Springer.

Twohig, M.P. (2008) *ACT Verbatim for Depression and Anxiety*. Oakland, CA: New Harbinger Publications.

10

ACT for Depression

Key Concepts

- From an ACT perspective, depression is believed to serve the function of helping the individual temporarily escape from difficult thoughts, feelings and memories.
- Suicidal ideation and behaviours commonly co-occur with depression, and the ACT model for depression can be readily applied to suicidal behaviours as well.
- Although an ACT approach for depression shares some features with behavioural activation, there are also distinct differences in the targets of these two treatments.

Depressive disorders are extremely common (Kessler et al., 2005), and major depressive disorder is one of the most significant causes of disability worldwide (Murray and Lopez, 1996). Several effective treatments for depression have been developed, including cognitive therapy (Beck et al., 1979) and behavioural activation (Martell et al., 2010). Acceptance and Commitment Therapy also has two studies that demonstrate that it is at least equivalent, if not superior, to cognitive therapy for depression, and that it works through different mechanisms (Zettle and Hayes, 1986; Zettle and Rains, 1989). For this reason, ACT is listed as an evidence-based treatment for depression with modest research support by Division 12 (Society of Clinical Psychology) of the American Psychological Association (see www.psychology.sunysb.edu/eklonsky-/division12/index).

USING ACT WITH DEPRESSION

The fact that ACT has been demonstrated to work through different mechanisms than cognitive therapy for depression is encouraging, because the case conceptualization for depression between the two treatment approaches is also fundamentally distinct. Within ACT, the case formulation is that affective disorders are the result of unsuccessful attempts to escape from challenging private events that the individual is unwilling to experience (Zettle, 2004). Extending from this model, anhedonia (the inability to take pleasure in activities one would usually find enjoyable), numbness and low energy all serve to provide a temporary escape function from unwanted feelings of disappointment, sadness, loss and guilt, as well as thoughts related to negative events in the past and negative evaluations of self. Although depression generally is associated with problems in living and functional impairments in the long run, it may in fact serve a useful function in the very short term. Thus, when conducting an analysis of the workability of depressive behaviours, the therapist must stay open to the possibility that depression may, in fact, have some 'benefits', in that it temporarily helps individuals to avoid their painful private experiences. However, as reviewed in Chapter 1, these escape and avoidance functions usually have negative consequences in the long term when they become the individual's characteristic way of responding to unwanted private events. Based on this conceptualization, the ACT therapist sets upon a course of work with the client around increasing willingness to experience the full spectrum of thoughts, feelings and other private events so that he does not need to resort to avoidance or escape.

Another component of the ACT conceptualization of depression involves fusion with negative cognitions about self or events that the client has experienced. A certain level of cognitive fusion is certainly normal for all language-capable humans. However, for those individuals who go on to meet the criteria for depression, there is a heightened tendency to fuse with and believe the thoughts that relate to one's negative judgements of one's self or thoughts that relate to negative experiences that are in the individual's history. Cognitive therapy models certainly also view negative cognitions as central to the conceptualization of depression. However, as has been pointed out throughout this text (and especially in Chapter 4), ACT uses defusion techniques rather than disputation or other strategies designed to change the content or response to these thoughts.

It is also important to note that individuals can even become fused with the label of depression. From an ACT model, depression is not something that one 'has'. It's not even something that one feels. Instead, depression is a label that is used to describe a broad-based dampening down of responses that functions to help the person escape private experiences that the individual evaluates as unwanted. The problem with a person fusing with the label of depression is that the client who does so is less likely to engage in new behaviours and is more likely to remain stuck, in order to maintain coherence between the label and her behaviour.

In order to assist with defusion from this, it can be helpful to return to the language conventions proposed in Chapter 4. For example, when the therapist notices that the client is stating that she is depressed, or that she couldn't follow through with a commitment due to her depression, the therapist would gently suggest that the client reframe this cognition as, 'I'm having the thought that I'm depressed', rather than 'I am depressed'. The first phrase non-judgementally describes a cognition, while the second phrase provides a core label for the overall individual. Similarly, the client who says, 'I can't make decisions due to chronic depression', would be asked to reframe this as, 'I'm having the thought that I am chronically depressed, and I choose not to make decisions'. This type of reframe works to identify thoughts as thoughts, rather than as reality, and puts the responsibility for acting or not acting on the individual, rather than on the 'depression'. As a means of shorthand, a therapist may describe someone as depressed in order to communicate and describe a certain set of characteristic behaviours. However, when an individual labels herself this way, it becomes much more problematic.

EMPIRICAL SUPPORT FOR ACT WITH DEPRESSION (SELECTED READINGS)

Forman, E.M., Herbert, J.D., Moitra, E., Yeomans, P.D. and Geller, P.A. (2007) A randomized controlled effectiveness trial of Acceptance and Commitment Therapy and Cognitive Therapy for anxiety and depression. *Behaviour Modification*, 31: 772–99.

Gaudiano, B.A., Miller, I.W. and Herbert, J.D. (2007) The treatment of psychotic major depression: is there a role for adjunctive psychotherapy? *Psychotherapy and Psychosomatics*, 76: 271–7.

Petersen, C.L. and Zettle, R.D. (2009) Treating inpatients with comorbid depression and alcohol use disorders: a comparison of Acceptance and Commitment Therapy and treatment as usual. *The Psychological Record*, 59: 521–36.

Zettle, R.D. and Hayes, S.C. (1986) Dysfunctional control by client verbal behaviour: the context of reason giving. *The Analysis of Verbal Behaviour*, 4: 30–8.

Zettle, R.D. and Rains, J.C. (1989) Group cognitive and contextual therapies in treatment of depression. *Journal of Clinical Psychology*, 45: 436–45.

Zettle, R.D., Rains, J.C. and Hayes, S.C. (in press) Processes of change in Acceptance and Commitment Therapy and Cognitive Therapy for depression: a mediational reanalysis of Zettle and Rains (1989). *Behaviour Modification*.

In addition to a focus on willingness and defusion, ACT work with depression also provides an opportunity to work with clients on present-moment awareness. The content that the depressed individual struggles and fuses with is frequently focused on things that have occurred in the past. For example, a depressed client who has had a significant personal loss in her life could spend hours of her waking time each day thinking about an individual who has died, reflecting on past events and ruminating on the circumstances of the individual's death. (This is in contrast with the focus of an individual with an anxiety disorder, who is much more likely to be fixated on potential events that may or may not occur in the future.) Thus, in ACT, it is essential to work with depressed clients on coming into contact with the present moment, rather than staying mired in the past. Practices that promote mindfulness of the here and now can be a powerful antidote to remaining stuck in days gone by and opportunities lost, once the client is open and willing to begin to move from the past into the present.

Clients who become depressed are often overly fused with certain aspects of the conceptualized self. In addition to a client simply describing herself by saying, 'I am chronically depressed', she may also become fused with a certain description or story that provides her with an analysis of why it is that she has become depressed. For this reason, ACT therapists will frequently target these stories that provide the client's internal explanations for depression. There is a difference between agreeing upon the facts of the situation and agreeing that the connections and implications that the client draws from those facts are 'true'. The ACT therapist will point out that the most dangerous thing about believing our own stories is that it can make our past into our future (Strosahl, 2004). If we believe the story to be the truth, then it constrains our current behaviour to fit the story and decreases the likelihood that we will try out new responses and strategies. The Life Story exercise below can thus be one approach to loosening the hold of the conceptualized self on current depressive behaviour (Zettle et al., 2009).

Life Story Exercise

In this exercise, the client is asked to begin by writing a one- or two-page narrative of the life events that have unfolded and conspired to lead the individual to become depressed. This is generally assigned as homework, although it can be done in the session if the client has significant problems with homework compliance. In the session after this assignment has been completed, the client is asked to read the life story narrative aloud to the therapist. At this time, the therapist may wish to make an internal note of any significant themes that have been brought up in the writing, as this provides good fodder for motifs to look for throughout therapy with this client. The client is then asked to go through the written product and underline those things that could be considered facts – that everyone could agree actually occurred. The therapist may need to assist with this at first, as some clients will think that everything they have written is an indisputable fact. The example below provides a condensed example of such a story:

> I grew up in Wales, the eldest daughter of four children. When I was 10 years old, my mother died suddenly in a car accident, and I was devastated. Because my father was a selfish bastard, he ignored my needs and just assumed that I would step into my mother's role, so all of the household and childcare responsibilities fell to me. I worked hard to take care of my brothers and my sister, but I was miserable inside. I think I started to become depressed basically the moment that my mom died. From that point on, I was never allowed to live the life of a normal child. I always had to be the caretaker. Finally, at the age of 18, I couldn't take it anymore, and I married a boy from the next town over, just so that I could escape the hell of my home. I haven't ever been happy in my marriage, and I have ended up being just as much of a caretaker for him and our three children as I was for my father and siblings. I don't see that there is any real way out of the situation that I'm in, and that hopelessness just makes me more and more depressed.

In this example, the therapist helps to identify those parts of the story that are irrefutable facts. These are generally the parts that describe overt behaviours or events that others could agree did occur. Descriptions of emotional states and all-or-nothing statements, such as 'I was never allowed to live the life of a normal child' or 'I wasn't ever happy in my marriage', cannot be considered facts, as other observers could potentially point out instances where these statements were factually incorrect. Similarly, statements about the cause of her depression or the probability of her recovery are verbal attributions, not observable facts. After going through this process with the client, the therapist would then request that the client rewrite the life story, so that it ends in some other way than with the client being depressed.

The therapist should make clear that it is not required that the new story have a happy ending. The goal is simply to demonstrate how these same facts could add up to a different result. For example, the client could have become riddled with guilt that she should have reminded her mother to be safe the morning that she was killed. Or she could have become highly anxious and never agreed to travel by car again. Or she could have gone on to become a safety advocate, championing new seat belt laws in her country. The client is asked to rewrite the story two or three times, each time using the same facts that were underlined in the first version, but tying them together in different ways and ending with a conclusion other than the client being depressed. The goal of the exercise is not to convince the client that she should not be depressed, but rather to help her defuse from this aspect of her conceptualized self and loosen up from the story that she has been holding on to as if it were the truth. The idea is that if she can see that her depression is not a foregone conclusion or a reason that her life cannot change, she may be able to begin to engage in more flexible and effective behaviour, rather than being defined by her conceptualized self and life story.

The final component of an ACT-based conceptualization of depression involves an analysis of withdrawal from values-based action. Individuals who are depressed frequently report low energy and loss of interest in things that previously had been enjoyable. They may often begin withdrawing from activities and situations in which they would have usually participated. Such withdrawal may initially occur in order to escape pain or protect oneself in the short term, but over time, it can significantly constrain behaviour and reduce the amount of natural reinforcement available in the individual's environment. This restriction on valued behaviour also means that not only is the client not moving forward with her life, but she is also not able to deal with current life problems directly. As Strosahl and Robinson (2008) have described this trade-off, the client can either manage her mood, or she can manage her life.

For these reasons, it is extremely important within the ACT model to work with the client to reconnect with her values and identify targets for building committed action. For some clients who have been depressed for a long span of time, the years of generalized dampening of responses may make it very difficult to connect with those things that are truly important and valued to them. The therapist can refer to the strategies for identifying values described in Chapter 7 to inform ways of working with clients to reconnect with their values. With a chronically depressed individual, it can also be useful to ask the client to go back to the last time in her life that she was not depressed. For example, the client whose life story is described above might be asked to try to recall what was important to her as a child before her mother was killed, as well as the dreams that she might have had for her life at that time. Although the specific goals that she had for her life at the age of 9 or 10 may or may not be achievable or relevant any longer, this work can help identify the values that she likely still has in place. It is more important to work with clients next to develop small, achievable goals that can be accomplished in the service of those values than to develop grand behavioural commitments. In order to break out of the cycle of depressed behaviour, it is most essential to have the client work on successive behaviours that are value-driven, such that she can begin to contact the naturally reinforcing properties of engaging in values-consistent behaviour within her environment.

USING ACT WITH SUICIDAL BEHAVIOURS

Consistent with the general ACT conceptualization of depression, suicidal ideation and other suicidal behaviours are also seen as a common experiential escape strategy. Because of the high frequency of suicidal behaviour in depressed individuals (Angst et al., 2002), therapists should routinely assess for suicidal thoughts and behaviours with all depressed clients. However, it is also important to note that suicidal thoughts and behaviours are quite common in general, regardless of whether someone meets the criteria for a psychiatric diagnosis or not (Chiles and Strosahl, 2004), and thus such an assessment is likely more broadly applicable. Individuals who have thoughts of killing themselves are sometimes overwhelmed and frightened by their own suicidal ideation. Thus, when the issue of suicide is brought up clinically, the ACT therapist has the opportunity to reframe suicidal ideation and suicidal behaviour as more examples of how the client has been trying to get rid of, change or control his emotions. Once clients have a new way of looking at these thoughts, it can be easier to defuse from them slightly and see them for what they are (the products of a mind looking for an escape route), rather than feeling like this is something external and mysterious that is happening to the client (Zettle, 2004). In addition, by providing clients with a meaningful way of understanding thoughts of suicide, when those thoughts next emerge, it can serve as a cue for clients to identify the thoughts and feelings that they are currently unwilling to have and then mindfully practise other strategies, such as defusion and willingness, to engage with those experiences.

Chiles and Strosahl (2004) identify that suicidal behaviour often serves both an instrumental and an expressive function, occurring when the client experiences private events that he views as intolerable, inescapable and interminable. Interpersonally, communicating that one is depressed or suicidal may also keep people from making demands on the depressed individual. Thus, suicidal behaviour may have short-term consequences that provide reinforcement for such behaviour. However, the ACT therapist is encouraged to work with the client to examine both the short- and long-term workability of engaging in suicidal behaviour (Strosahl, 2004). Although suicidal thoughts and behaviour may work temporarily to provide relief from ongoing, uncomfortable private events, this pattern of behaviour generally leads to disconnection from valued living in a variety of domains. In addition, if the client follows through on the ultimate escape strategy of committing suicide, then he permanently loses the opportunity to improve his life and move forward with what is important to him.

Because suicidal ideation is simply part of the common human experience, the goal of ACT cannot be the elimination of suicidal thoughts and behaviours entirely. Instead, the ACT therapist must learn to be accepting of the fact that clients will sometimes experience suicidal ideation and to be able to sit non-judgementally with the client when this does occur. This is not to minimize the magnitude of the problem of suicide. Certainly, clients do kill themselves, and this is a tragic outcome to be avoided to the highest possible extent. However, if the therapist balks and drops everything to deviate from the ACT treatment model each time the client becomes suicidal, this just reinforces the escape function of the behaviour and takes the client off track. The ACT therapist must find the balance between validating the client's desire to escape from the current pain, while coming down firmly on the side of life (Strosahl, 2004). (For a more comprehensive model describing practical strategies for managing suicidal risk within an ACT-consistent framework, please see Chiles and Strosahl [2004].)

CONSIDERATIONS IN USING ACT WITH DEPRESSION

Because of the shared focus on increasing follow-through with committed behaviour, many therapists wonder about the similarities and differences between ACT and behavioural activation (Martell et al., 2010) for depression. A basic analysis demonstrates that both approaches underscore a focus on committed action, and both therapies endeavour to get people in touch with the reinforcing qualities (e.g. a sense of completion and satisfaction, natural social contingencies) of taking action. However, behavioural activation does not include an emphasis on those actions being directed by the client's values, and only ACT includes the focus on defusion, willingness and self-as-context (Zettle, 2007). Although behavioural activation does not explicitly teach mindfulness, it does suggest that 'attending to experience' is a strategy that can be practised as an alternative to rumination (Martell et al., 2001). Thus, the theories and methods of behavioural activation and ACT are certainly consistent with one another; however, the rationale for engaging in committed action and the centrality of behavioural action in each approach is slightly different. (For a further analysis of the similarities and differences between these two behavioural treatments, see Kanter et al. [2006].)

As was described in Chapter 8, it is useful to look for potential barriers to clients being willing to move forward with their lives, and this is certainly true when working with depressed individuals. Many depressed clients have become invested not just in their story of what has led to their depression, but also in fulfilling the role of the 'martyr' (Zettle, 2004). For those clients who see suffering as part of their identity (see the life story above as one example), it can be difficult to let the martyr status go, in the service of moving forward with life. Similarly, for those individuals who have been wronged or truly harmed by others, it can also be extremely difficult to let go of what may be very valid resentments that have defined the client's identity and major life choices over time. For this reason, Strosahl (2004) has conceptualized forgiveness as an act of willingness. From an ACT perspective, the goal of forgiveness is not to forget what happened or imply that what has happened was good or right. However, if the client is living her life in order to prove that she was wronged by a specific person or by life circumstances, then she can't live her life in a way that moves it forward in the service of her values. Choosing forgiveness is about setting yourself free, so that you can move on with your own life.

As implied throughout this chapter, it takes strong clinical skills to be able to work on these issues with depressed clients without invalidating their very real experiences and losses. None of this work can be done without first building a trusting, compassionate therapeutic relationship. Compassion does not always mean being soft though. The ACT therapist can demonstrate immense compassion for the client by always bringing choices back to workability and demonstrating that the most important thing is helping the client to move on from her suffering and reclaim her life now!

Summary

The ACT model conceptualizes both depression and suicidal behaviours as serving to help an individual escape from private events that are painful or aversive. However, when this strategy becomes the characteristic way that the individual interacts with the environment, it can lead to notable constrictions on values-based behaviour. When working with depressed clients, the ACT therapist uses all of the core processes of ACT to help the client come into contact with the present, defuse from thoughts and conceptions that are not helpful, increase willingness to experience the full range of private events and re-engage with valued living.

Points for Review and Reflection

- Describe how the ACT conceptualization of depression indicates a focus on each of the ACT core processes: willingness, defusion, present-moment awareness, self-as-context, values and committed action.
- What is the goal of the Life Story exercise? How would you approach this exercise with clients so that they would not feel invalidated by the suggestion that their lives could possibly be different?
- Try the life story exercise for yourself. What do you notice about that experience?
- Describe two differences between the practices of ACT and behavioural activation for depression.

Further Reading

Chiles, J. and Strosahl, K. (2004) *Handbook for the Clinical Assessment and Treatment of the Suicidal Patient*. Washington, DC: American Psychiatric Press.

(Continued)

(Continued)

Kanter, J.W., Baruch, D.E. and Gaynor, S.T. (2006) Acceptance and Commitment Therapy and behavioural activation for the treatment of depression: description and comparison. *The Behaviour Analyst*, 29: 161–85.

Strosahl, K.D. and Robinson, P. J. (2008) *The Mindfulness and Acceptance Workbook for Depression: Using Acceptance and Commitment Therapy to Move through Depression and Create a Life Worth Living*. Oakland, CA: New Harbinger Publications.

Twohig, M.P. (2008) *ACT Verbatim for Depression and Anxiety*. Oakland, CA: New Harbinger Publications.

Zettle, R.D. (2007) *ACT for Depression: A Clinician's Guide to Using Acceptance and Commitment Therapy in Treating Depression*. Oakland, CA: New Harbinger Publications.

11

ACT for Substance Use and Addictive Disorders

> ## Key Concepts
>
> - Problematic substance use behaviours can be conceptualized within a framework of experiential avoidance.
> - The ACT approach to the treatment of substance abuse focuses less on abstinence or substance use reduction as goals unto themselves, and more on how to return the client to a present-moment focus that allows for committed action based on the client's values.
> - ACT can facilitate the treatment of substance use that is comorbid with anxiety, depression or a myriad of other problems, because each of these problems can be seen together as experiential avoidance disorders, rather than as distinct problems requiring separate interventions.

As with the other disorders highlighted in this text, substance use disorders are highly prevalent and can be conceptualized easily within an experiential avoidance framework. There is a growing body of evidence that suggests that individuals use substances as a way to try to regulate negative private events and that substance abuse is frequently a form of emotional avoidance, especially for those with high levels of anxiety symptoms (e.g. Armeli et al., 2003; Bonn-Miller et al., 2010; Stewart and Zeitlin, 1995). Although initial forays into substance use by some individuals may be primarily related to attempts to chase positive mood states, by the time that people present for treatment in a clinical setting, this balance has often tipped more significantly toward avoiding negative private events.

In addition to evidence that substance use is correlated with experiential avoidance (Forsyth et al., 2003), multiple treatment studies also reinforce the applicability of an ACT approach to this class of clinical problems. In one of the largest-scale ACT outcome studies with substance abuse, ACT was found to be effective in the treatment of polysubstance-abusing opiate addicts on methadone at six-month follow-up (Hayes et al., 2004a). Results of case studies also suggest that ACT may be effective for methadone detoxification (Stotts et al., 2009) and for the treatment of marijuana dependence (Twohig et al., 2007) and alcohol dependence (Heffner et al., 2003) in adults. Further, clinical trials have also demonstrated that ACT is superior to two empirically supported treatments for smoking cessation – nicotine replacement therapy and CBT (Gifford et al., 2004; Hernandez-Lopez et al., 2009). Finally, preliminary data show that an ACT-based professional training workshop has promise for the reduction of burnout and stigmatizing attitudes toward substance abusers in substance abuse counsellors (Hayes et al., 2004b). In summary, multiple sources of data suggest that ACT is appropriate and effective for the treatment of addictive disorders and that experiential avoidance is a core problem for this class of behaviours.

USING ACT WITH SUBSTANCE USE DISORDERS

As with most any treatment approach, the opening phase of treatment for ACT with substance use disorders begins with assessment. The initial stage of assessment not only provides the information that will be used to identify a treatment plan, but also begins the development of a therapeutic relationship. Because substance use disorders are among the most stigmatized of all mental health conditions (Corrigan et al., 2000), clients presenting for substance use treatment are likely to have had negative interactions with multiple people (including treatment providers) related to their addictive behaviour in the past. Thus, from the initial interactions, the ACT therapist has an opportunity to begin this relationship in a novel way for the client. It is important that in both verbal and non-verbal communication, the ACT therapist communicate a stance of non-judgementality and willingness to allow the client to identify what is most important to work on in treatment. These characteristics can be conveyed both in the types of questions asked and the ways in which questions are posed to the client. The job of the ACT therapist is not to coerce or convince the client to make changes or to stop using substances, but to focus on workability and supporting the client in creating a life that is more meaningful. By attending to this therapeutic stance, starting with the beginning stages of assessment, the client and therapist have an opportunity to begin the hard work ahead in a collaborative and effective manner.

This assessment includes not just quantity and frequency of substance abuse, and levels of experiential avoidance on standardized measures, but also a careful assessment of substance abuse history and the costs that this behaviour has had in multiple valued domains (Wilson and Byrd, 2004). While assessing the history of the use of different substances, it can be useful to notice shifts in quantity, frequency or type of substance used and to determine if there were concomitant changes in levels of avoidance or willingness in the client's life at those times. The client may also be asked to provide specific examples of how substance use has affected his life in each of the domains of valued living described in Chapter 7. This is done not for the sake of wallowing in the losses that the client has experienced or the ineffective decisions he has made, but to lay the groundwork for Creative Hopelessness and its analysis of the workability of using substances and other methods of avoidance. Specific assessment handouts for these purposes can be found in Wilson and Byrd (2004).

After respectfully conducting this assessment process, the therapist will frequently move into the process of engendering a state of Creative Hopelessness. During this shift, it is important to recognize that although substance use encompasses a large class of behaviours that can be conceptualized as avoidance, it is certainly not the only type of clinically relevant behaviour that will be in the client's avoidant repertoire. When beginning this stage of treatment, it can be useful to ask the client to generate a list of the major things that he is struggling with and trying to change. This could include problems with relationships and loss, problems with mood and anxiety, feelings of rejection or isolation, substance use, and a variety of other items. After generating this list, the next step is to say something like: 'It sounds like you've been struggling with these issues for quite a long time and have tried a variety of things to get them to change. What I don't want us to do is to keep doing the things that haven't worked, so I wonder if we can brainstorm a bit and see if we can identify all the strategies that you've tried over the years to deal with these things you've been struggling with'. Below is one list of attempted strategies generated (with the assistance of a therapist) by a middle-aged man who had entered treatment with a 30-year history of alcohol and heroin use:

- Medications and methadone
- Drugs
- Alcohol
- Isolation
- Sleep
- Sex
- Reading
- Staying busy with activities
- Pushing people away with anger
- Therapy
- Overeating

- Just toughing it out
- Stuffing emotions
- Distancing myself from people and situations
- Geographical solutions (moving away)
- Overworking.

This list was generated between client and therapist over the course of only about 5–10 minutes, and obviously each client will produce a somewhat different set of examples, depending on his life experiences. Such a list can also be generated in the context of group treatment for addictive disorders. In both contexts, the therapist can approach this in a curious and enthusiastic way, rather than by being negative and pessimistic. By approaching this work with a sense of curiosity (this can be framed as being almost like a detective), the therapist helps to defuse and lighten what can otherwise be very heavy work, in the service of helping the client to see that there are multiple ways of approaching these issues.

The next step is then working with the client (or the group) to identify the theme or similarity that ties these strategies together. The therapist can say something to the effect of: 'Well, as I said, we want to make sure as we move forward that we're not simply doing the same things you've already tried, because if they were going to work, they would have worked already. But as I look at this list, it's pretty long, and it would be hard to keep track of each one of these things separately. So, I wonder if we can take a look at the list again and see if there is something that ties them together, maybe like a theme? Because if we can identify what they have in common, then that will give us a really solid place to start'. When presented with a list like this, clients will generally be able to come up with something like:

> It's a series of things that haven't worked. Or, I guess, they work in the short term, but they haven't done me any good in the long run.

> It's a bunch of things that I've tried just to get by, but they haven't really addressed the actual problem, and have probably just made things worse.

Depending on what the client brings up, the therapist can provide some other inputs, suggesting that maybe these items can be seen as attempts at control, avoidance or trying to get away from pain and difficult experiences. The specific word or phrase that is settled on is not what's important. What is important is finding a theme that resonates with the client, depending on the type of language that he uses. The client must be able to connect with the experience of the futility of these strategies and have some way of categorizing them that works for him. This process is exceptionally important with this group of clients, in order to reinforce the focus on workability and to set up the hard work of willingness. The client must personally contact the futility of the control agenda if he is to consider trying something new. While conducting this work, the therapist should also try to assess the extent to which the client thinks that substance use does actually work to eliminate or control private events.

EMPIRICAL SUPPORT FOR ACT WITH SUBSTANCE USE AND ADDICTIVE DISORDERS (SELECTED READINGS)

Batten, S.V., DeViva, J.C., Santanello, A.P., Morris, L.J., Benson, P.R. and Mann, M.A. (2009) Acceptance and Commitment Therapy for comorbid PTSD and substance use disorders. In J. Blackledge, J. Ciarrochi and F. Dean (eds), *Acceptance and Commitment Therapy: Current Directions* (pp. 311–28). Queensland, Australia: Australian Academic Press.

Gifford, E.V., Kohlenberg, B.S., Hayes, S.C., Antonuccio, D.O., Piasecki, M.M., Rasmussen-Hall, M.L. and Palm, K.M. (2004) Acceptance-based treatment for smoking cessation. *Behaviour Therapy*, 35: 689–705.

Hayes, S.C., Bissett, R., Roget, N., Padilla, M., Kohlenberg, B.S., Fisher, G., Masuda, A., Pistorello, J., Rye, A.K., Berry, K. and Niccolls, R. (2004a) The impact of Acceptance and Commitment Training and multicultural training on the stigmatizing attitudes and professional burnout of substance abuse counselors. *Behaviour Therapy*, 35: 821–35.

Hayes, S.C., Wilson, K.G., Gifford, E.V., Bissett, R.T., Piasecki, M., Batten, S.V., Byrd, M.R. and Gregg, J. (2004b) A preliminary trial of twelve-step facilitation and acceptance and commitment therapy with polysubstance-abusing methadone-maintained opiate addicts. *Behaviour Therapy*, 35: 667–88.

Heffner, M., Eifert, G.H., Parker, B.T., Hernandez, D.H. and Sperry, J.A. (2003) Valued directions: Acceptance and Commitment Therapy in the treatment of alcohol dependence. *Cognitive and Behavioural Practice*, 10: 378–83.

Hernandez-Lopez, M., Luciano, M.C., Bricker, J.B., Roales-Nieto, J.G. and Montesinos, F. (2009) Acceptance and Commitment Therapy for smoking cessation: a preliminary study of its effectiveness in comparison with cognitive behavioural therapy. *Psychology of Addictive Behaviours*, 23: 723–30.

Luoma, J.B., Kohlenberg, B.S., Hayes, S.C., Bunting, K. and Rye, A.K. (2008) Reducing self-stigma in substance abuse through Acceptance and Commitment Therapy: model, manual development, and pilot outcomes. *Addiction Research and Theory*, 16: 149–65.

Twohig, M.P., Shoenberger, D. and Hayes, S.C. (2007) A preliminary investigation of Acceptance and Commitment Therapy as a treatment for marijuana dependence in adults. *Journal of Applied Behaviour Analysis*, 40: 619–32.

Through a variety of means of avoidance, chronic substance abusers have made it a way of life to do anything they can to get out of the present moment, and the immediate reinforcement that escape or avoidance through substance use provides can be powerful. Thus, a focus on mindfulness is essential. Many substance use treatment protocols in ACT include a mindfulness exercise in each session, to ensure that the client gains these skills in his repertoire. Only in the present moment can one begin to move toward what is important instead of away from pain, disappointment and other difficult private events.

Over time, the level of behavioural constriction in the lives of substance abusers takes on great magnitude. Life becomes much more about seeking and using substances, getting away from the present moment, and less about connecting with individuals and activities that are important to the person. ACT can work on both reducing the avoidance associated with the substance abuse and increasing values-driven behaviour. Individuals with a lengthy substance abuse history have often negated their own values for years at a time. It is painful to then try to reconnect with those values, because the client must come into contact with all that has been lost and all of the times where he didn't act in accordance with those values. Thus, the values work can be both very hopeful (it is a new way of looking at things that isn't just focused on abstinence) and also very painful. It is essential that the therapist reinforce that she is 100 per cent committed to working with the client on these important things, regardless of how hard it gets. Issues of the sequencing of values work within treatment and the importance of focusing on values for those who are court-ordered or otherwise mandated to treatment covered in Chapter 7 are extremely relevant for this population.

As mentioned previously, the focus of ACT with this population is not directly on abstinence or even necessarily on reducing substance use, and the ACT therapist cannot be personally invested in reduced substance use or abstinence as the outcome. The focus is on living a life that the client values; however, many times, the client will identify that continuing to use substances is inconsistent with those values (Heffner et al., 2003). It can be very useful for the therapist to know to what degree the client actually sees a discrepancy between valued life directions and current substance use behaviours. If the client does self-identify that he wishes to stop drinking, using drugs, smoking, etc., then the therapist will work with the client on both identifying valued directions and goals, and then making behavioural commitments to move forward in these areas. It is essential that the therapist learn to respond in a non-judgemental manner, regardless of whether or not the client reaches the target commitments in a given week. For example, the client needs to be able to trust that the therapist will be there and will remain committed to the work, even if the client does not meet a commitment in the service of reduced substance use one week. This is communicated directly ahead of time by the therapist, but the therapist also needs to be able to demonstrate this absolute level of acceptance and compassion in the session as well.

Over time, ACT therapists generally realize that they don't have control over the client's behaviour anyway, and so it may become more natural to respond in this way to slips and relapses. However, what may not be so apparent is that the other side of the coin is true as well. That is, the therapist also needs to learn not to respond in an overly excited or enthusiastic way when the client does keep a behavioural goal of sobriety or anything else. It is certainly natural to want to celebrate success with the client in an attempt to share the experience and reinforce the client's more functional behaviour. However, if the therapist says verbally that the client's abstinence is not what is most important, but is then enthusiastically positive when the client keeps a commitment to abstinence, it will not take long for the client to be able to realize that the therapist is not nearly so pleased or even neutral when the target commitment is not kept. The ACT therapist must find the balance of staying engaged and genuine and, at the same time, not giving implicit messages that she is passing judgement or giving approval if the client does or does not follow-through with a commitment. The therapist must remember that this is the client's life that is being worked on, and only the client can decide what is workable for him.

One way to divert from a sole focus on abstinence-based goals is by choosing more vital goals than simply 'not smoking/drinking/using drugs this week'. In the first place, this is a goal that a dead man could achieve (Lindsley, 1968), and thus not a goal filled with vitality and purpose. Instead, the individual could choose goals that are about moving valued areas of his life forward. Or, if the client truly wants to choose a goal focused on the substance use itself, then the therapist might suggest that the client choose to use or not use mindfully each time there is an urge to engage in the behaviour. For example, the client could be asked to notice each time there is an urge and to spend two or three minutes simply being mindful of all of the thoughts, feelings, memories, bodily sensations and urges that arise. The client can then be asked to spend two or three minutes focusing on values and what is important to him in his life, before he mindfully makes a choice of whether or not to smoke, drink or use. This is an in vivo version of the imaginal exercise of 'Pausing in the Moment' described in Chapter 8 and shares some characteristics with techniques such as 'urge surfing' (Marlatt and Witkiewitz, 2005) and the 'three-minute breathing space' (Williams et al., 2007). This mindful, present-moment focus is in direct contrast to the way in which clients generally experience the initial choices to use, often described as being on 'auto-pilot'. Clients who practise such an exercise will often return to the next week's session with a statement such as, 'You ruined my high!' Indeed, it is difficult to retain the same amount of relief or pleasure from problematic use when the individual is fully present and focused on values.

CONSIDERATIONS IN USING ACT WITH SUBSTANCE USE DISORDERS

Working with substance-abusing clients is challenging, rewarding and at times very frustrating for even the most seasoned and accepting therapist. The therapist must recognize the relapsing nature of these problems and accept that slips are simply part of the process of growing and sequentially building patterns of committed action in the service of values. It is important for client and therapist to both remember that if the client slips on a behavioural goal related to substance use that this should not be taken as an excuse for the client to give up or spiral downward. Instead, the client then has the opportunity to notice where he is, pick himself up again and immediately begin moving forward with making, breaking and eventually keeping commitments to valued directions and goals. Even if the client shows up for the session under the influence of substances, as long as he is not so inebriated as to be unable to engage productively with the work of the session at all, this can be a productive moment to work together on contacting the costs of using and recommitting to healthier choices in the service of the client's values.

One point that is notable about the ACT approach to substance abuse treatment is that it need not occur in isolation from treatment of other co-occurring problems. In most cases, treatment systems are set up such that substance abuse treatment programmes and other mental health treatment programmes are organized and delivered separately. This may be due to the vagaries of funding sources, training systems, diagnostic nomenclature and even stigmatizing attitudes on the part of mental health professionals. However, when one truly examines such a model, it becomes obvious that the client with two or three co-occurring disorders is simply one person whose functioning cannot be meaningfully carved up into the substance abusing part and the part with mental health concerns. Thus, it is important not to focus just on substance use disorders, but also on the ways in which substance use intersects with other comorbid problems.

This ability to conceptualize behavioural problems based on transdiagnostic functional dimensions and processes such as experiential avoidance is one of the strengths of an ACT approach. Because many other conditions can be conceptualized with the same experiential avoidance framework as can substance use disorders, when these types of problems co-occur, the ACT therapist can work with them all within a consistent model. In fact, preliminary evidence from existing ACT treatment studies does demonstrate that comorbid substance use disorders can be treated effectively alongside post-traumatic stress disorder, depression and personality disorders (Batten et al., 2009; Batten and Hayes, 2005; Hayes et al., 2004a; Petersen and Zettle, 2009). Such an integrated model is truly innovative in that it allows the therapist to conceptualize a variety of comorbid concerns based on their overlapping problems with avoidance, rather than having to view them as entirely separate diagnoses that would require completely distinct treatments.

Before conducting ACT with substance use disorders, it can be helpful for the therapist to consider the compatibility of ACT with one of the most widely used approaches to dealing with alcoholism and addictive disorders in the community: the 12-step model. Such an analysis will likely demonstrate that while there may be different areas of emphasis between the two approaches, the two share many concepts and principles with one another (Batten et al., 2009; Wilson et al., 2000). For example, the ACT focus on workability is very consistent with the 12-step concept of examining whether one's life is unmanageable or out of control. Further, the 12-step acknowledgement of 'powerlessness' is not unlike coming to a state of Creative Hopelessness early on in ACT. In addition, both approaches encourage individuals to identify those things that are most important in their lives and to take specific actions to move in those directions. The words of the 'Serenity Prayer', regularly used in 12-step approaches, also have a clear resonance within ACT. The ACT therapist who is well informed about the 12-step model will have another tool in her repertoire for effectively facilitating client behaviour change related to substance use disorders.

As a reminder, the ACT therapist should not underestimate the power of choosing a therapeutic stance that is non-judgemental and agnostic about whether or not individuals should be using substances. Such a humane, non-stigmatizing approach is vastly different from the way in which the community and even other health care professionals often approach individuals who have problems with substance misuse. When clients learn that they can be honest about their substance use and that the therapeutic relationship will remain consistent and supportive regardless, it allows them to open up and engage with the relevant issues in a new and more productive way. The ACT therapist's focus on values as defined by the client, rather than on socially defined norms about substance use, allows the therapist to work side by side with the client rather than on opposing sides from one another. This accepting interpersonal stance also models for the client the relationship that he could potentially have with himself if he could stop judging himself for his substance use and other 'failures' and instead focus on acceptance, willingness and moving forward with his life.

Summary

ACT provides a novel way of approaching the treatment of substance abuse and addictive disorders, whether the target substance is a drug, a glass of alcohol or a cigarette. The experience of reducing or ceasing substance use will inevitably be accompanied by uncomfortable bodily sensations and other difficult private events. Thus, ACT focuses on a willing stance toward these

(Continued)

(Continued)

experiences, while choosing mindful contact with the present moment, so that the individual can move forward and reclaim a life full of things that she values.

Points for Review and Reflection

- Describe several avoidance strategies that substance users may be likely to have utilized in addition to the substance abuse itself.
- Why doesn't an ACT treatment approach for substance use disorders stress the importance of abstinence or substance use moderation? What treatment targets are stressed instead?
- What is the benefit of using an ACT model to treat substance use disorders that are comorbid with other psychological conditions?

Further Reading

Batten, S.V., DeViva, J.C., Santanello, A.P., Morris, L.J., Benson, P.R. and Mann, M.A. (2009) Acceptance and Commitment Therapy for comorbid PTSD and substance use disorders. In J. Blackledge, J. Ciarrochi, and F. Dean (eds), *Acceptance and Commitment Therapy: Current Directions* (pp. 311–28). Queensland, Australia: Australian Academic Press.

Hayes, S.C., Wilson, K.G., Gifford, E.V., Bissett, R.T., Piasecki, M., Batten, S.V., Byrd, M.R. and Gregg, J. (2004) A preliminary trial of twelve-step facilitation and Acceptance and Commitment Therapy with polysubstance-abusing methadone-maintained opiate addicts. *Behaviour Therapy*, 35: 667–88.

Hernandez-Lopez, M., Luciano, M.C., Bricker, J.B., Roales-Nieto, J.G. and Montesinos, F. (2009) Acceptance and Commitment Therapy for smoking cessation: a preliminary study of its effectiveness in comparison with cognitive behavioural therapy. *Psychology of Addictive Behaviours*, 23: 723–30.

Wilson, K.G. and Byrd, M.R. (2004) ACT for substance abuse and dependence. In S.C. Hayes and K.D. Strosahl (eds), *A Practical Guide to Acceptance and Commitment Therapy* (pp. 153–84). New York: Springer.

Wilson, K.G., Hayes, S.C. and Byrd, M.R. (2000) Exploring compatibilities between Acceptance and Commitment Therapy and 12-step treatment for substance abuse. *Journal of Rational-Emotive Behaviour Therapy*, 18: 209–34.

12

Special Considerations in Applying ACT

Key Concepts

- ACT is an innovative contextual behavioural psychotherapy that focuses on pragmatism and workability across six core processes: Acceptance, Defusion, Contact with the Present Moment, Self-as-Context, Values and Committed Action.
- This approach to treatment has a strong theoretical basis and multiple sources of empirical evidence for its efficacy across a broad spectrum of disorders and problems in living.
- There are a variety of methods for interested therapists to continue to develop ACT core competences, including further reading, demonstration videos, participating in the online community of ACT practitioners and supervised clinical practice and consultation.

As described throughout this text, Acceptance and Commitment Therapy is a contextual behavioural approach to psychotherapy that builds upon several decades of theoretical and empirical work by its founder, Steve Hayes, and now many others around the world. This strong focus on the theoretical underpinnings of a treatment is somewhat unusual in a field that is generally marked by assembling a series of techniques that may be loosely organized around an untested theory. Although some practitioners may not be accustomed to such a strong emphasis on a theoretical model for clinical practice, it can be argued that having a coherent theory to undergird the work that occurs inside the therapy room can both enhance innovation and allow the therapist to respond to unexpected circumstances in a theoretically consistent way, even when faced with novel clinical experiences. Although ACT certainly has its share of unique techniques and tools, none of those specific tools is essential to the treatment in and of itself. Certainly, the hope is that the practical metaphors and exercises that have been provided in this text will be of use to the practitioner who is learning to implement ACT. However, it is also possible that one could conduct a course of therapy that is entirely ACT consistent without using any of the specific metaphors and tools described in this book. The theory behind ACT is its most central feature, and it is the resulting flexibility that has allowed ACT to be adapted across cultures, languages and presenting problems internationally.

A REVIEW OF CORE ACT PRINCIPLES AND PROCESSES

Within ACT, there are several core principles that underlie the work that is to be done. Because of its broad-based applicability, the main ideas within ACT can be applied to a wide variety of presenting problems that bring individuals to the therapy room. One of the principles that allows for such flexibility is ACT's focus on pragmatism and workability. In plain terms, this means that the client's values are what determine the targets of treatment. The ACT therapist's job is never to judge whether or not a client's behaviours or choices are problematic. The marker of whether or not something in the client's life is a problem is the client's own determination of whether it is bringing him closer to or further from what is important to him and what he wants his life to stand for. This freedom from preconceived judgements or assumptions allows the therapist to truly work alongside the client. The ACT therapist does not simply settle for a reduction in symptoms as a marker of therapeutic success. Success is determined by the client's ability to live a life that he values, undaunted by fleeting thoughts, feelings, bodily sensations or even circumstances, because even in the most trying of circumstances, individuals can choose to live by their own values. ACT therapists have the honour and opportunity to assist their clients in reconnecting with those core values in order to live a more meaningful life.

As described earlier, the ACT therapist's role is that of coach, advisor and witness, but not of expert or guru. The ACT model is crystal clear in its analysis that the issues that bring clients to psychotherapy are simply variants on the struggles that all humans face (and this includes therapists!). The ACT therapist should thus face this work with humility, humanity, genuineness and radical respect for the client's values and experiences. Many therapists who are new to the ACT approach report that it is a relief not to have to pretend to have all the answers in a session. Instead, the ACT therapist works along with the client to identify strategies for the way ahead, based on the core ACT theoretical framework.

This core framework consists of six basic processes: Acceptance, Defusion, Contact with the Present Moment, Self-as-Context, Values and Committed Action. Acceptance and Defusion are processes that allow the client to approach all manner of thoughts, feelings and private events from a stance that sees these private events for what they are – not what they say they are. Contact with the Present Moment and Self-as-Context provide the space and perspective that make it safe for the client to experience whatever private events may emerge, without having to struggle with or avoid the experience. Finally, Values and Committed Action provide the compass bearing and fuel for the client to be able to move forward in his life in a way that is meaningful for him.

Although the ACT model can be boiled down to a handful of core principles and processes, it is impossible to cover every facet of the model in one brief text. This book has been successful if it has done the following: explained the underlying theoretical model, summarized and referenced enough of the empirical literature so that it is clear that this work rests on a solid research base, presented the essentials of the general clinical approach and given examples of the techniques used in each component of ACT. By the end of this text, the reader should know whether this is a model that has resonance for him or her as a therapist. In hopes that this framework has connected with the reader, the chapter will end with suggestions for how to move to the next stage of ACT learning and training.

THE IMPORTANCE OF ASSESSMENT AND CASE CONCEPTUALIZATION

Although this text has focused primarily on the intervention components of ACT, it should be noted that effective ACT treatment rests on the bedrock of a solid initial assessment and case conceptualization. Assessment within ACT may be informal, such as the assessment of the client's avoidance strategies, or formal, such as a standardized measure of experiential avoidance like the Acceptance and Action Questionnaire (AAQ) (Hayes et al., 2004c). Further, some processes, such as values, can be assessed with either an informal or formal method of measurement. One of the shared values within the community of ACT practitioners and researchers is that such tools should not be considered proprietary and should be made as widely available as possible. Thus, measures such as the AAQ and a variety of values assessment handouts and metrics are available free of charge at www.contextualpsychology.org. Although not central to the ACT model, therapists may also choose to use traditional measures of symptomatology as another source of information about a given client's functioning.

Overall, the ACT therapist is committed to routine, ongoing assessment as a way of tracking progress, informing a case conceptualization and guiding individualized treatment efforts. In addition to structured assessments, the ACT therapist works to generate an evolving functional assessment of the client's behaviour and presenting problems in order to inform the course of treatment. To enhance these processes, ACT therapists also regularly use simple but effective modes of self-monitoring by the client, including diary cards, checklists, event logs and other ways of recording clinically relevant processes and behaviours in an individualized fashion (Bach and Moran, 2008). Many case conceptualization tools are available in print (Bach and Moran, 2008; Luoma et al., 2007) and online to assist the ACT therapist with identifying the most relevant targets for treatment across the six ACT core processes.

Overall, case conceptualization can be seen as comprising multiple domains: (1) information regarding the client's current presenting problems; (2) an analysis of the past situations that may have shaped the client's current problems; (3) a review of the current situations and circumstances that maintain the current problems; (4) a specification of the short- and long-term goals for therapy; and (5) details of an evidence-based treatment plan to address the issues identified above (Bach and Moran, 2008). An ACT-inspired case conceptualization is designed to be more focused on cross-cutting, functional dimensions such as experiential avoidance and cognitive fusion, rather than specific symptoms or diagnostic profiles. Those dimensions are guided by the six core ACT processes, each of which can cause significant problems in living when they contribute to psychological inflexibility rather than flexibility.

SEQUENCING ACT INTERVENTIONS

As mentioned early in this volume, there is no one particular sequence in which ACT concepts must be delivered. Even though many therapist manuals and treatment protocols may present the processes in the sequence in which they are described here, there is a distinct amount of variability in how the ACT tools and processes are presented and delivered across settings, presenting problems and therapists. There are yet no data to inform the question of whether it matters in which order the primary ACT concepts are presented. As mentioned earlier, the more competent and flexible an ACT therapist becomes, the less discrete the six processes may appear in a given course of treatment or even within a given session. Sometimes it may be clear from the individualized case conceptualization which treatment targets are primary and should be addressed first, but at other times, the course is not so apparent.

One heuristic that may be helpful to newer ACT therapists is the following: for clients who present to treatment with significant levels of distress, appear tired of the struggle or who clearly state that they wish to change something in their lives, the therapist may wish to begin with Creative Hopelessness and present the core ACT processes in approximately the order in which they are outlined in this book. For clients who do not present with any immediate distress, appear emotionally shut down, don't see any negative consequences for avoidance or are in treatment mandatorily, the therapist may wish to begin work with values and committed action. In this case, if avoidance or fusion is a significant problem, it will show itself to be a barrier to moving forward with actions soon enough, and then the other processes of ACT can be engaged. Regardless of the sequence in which these concepts are presented, the basic question to the client is: 'Could you choose to be willing to try something different if it would mean that your life could move forward in a way that means something to you?'

In addition to sequence, the beginning ACT therapist may also wonder how to know when to present one metaphor or exercise over another in a therapy session. It is important to note that a multitude of ACT-consistent exercises and metaphors are described in this text and in several others. The ACT therapist should not feel compelled to cover every one of these metaphors or experiential exercises with every client. In fact, it may be much more useful to choose a few representative metaphors that seem to resonate with the client that can be referred to over and over as a form of shorthand within the therapeutic dyad. Rigidly sticking to a defined set of interventions is likely to function more to unnecessarily increase the therapist's comfort than to actually address the needs of the individual client. The ACT therapist should be encouraged to try a variety of metaphors and interventions over time, and even to create novel, ACT-consistent metaphors that are designed to meet the needs and interests of a given client or set of clients. The primary reason that metaphors are proposed to be efficacious within ACT is because they call to mind concepts that are already familiar to the client and further apply them to the world of private events and behaviour. Thus, if the therapist truly understands the principles behind ACT and can create metaphors that resonate with the client's lived experience (e.g. sporting metaphors for the athlete, building metaphors for the carpenter), these metaphors will be likely to have more significance, tenacity and impact for the client.

TERMINATION FROM AN ACT PERSPECTIVE

Just as important as determining how to begin and to structure ACT treatment with a given client is the careful analysis of how and when to end a course of treatment. As described in Chapter 3, it is very useful to begin efforts with the client by agreeing to work together for a certain number of sessions and then to reassess progress toward the client's values at that time. Therapist and client can always agree to continue therapy for another period of time (assuming this is logistically possible), but it is important that this is done purposefully and mindfully, rather than simply staying in treatment together out of comfort or inertia. Frequently, clients and therapists alike may avoid a direct discussion of termination, because it can be awkward, difficult or painful. However, from an ACT perspective, the concept of ending therapy should be present from the very moment that therapy begins. Because both therapist and client know that this work is time-limited and focused on specific priority areas, they can remain more easily trained on the prize of therapy: the client learning how to move his own life forward, both currently and in the future.

Furthermore, it is important that the client not become overly reliant on the therapist, and instead that both client and therapist are carefully focused on ensuring that the client is constantly adding new skills to his repertoire that he can use even once therapy is complete. Although the therapeutic philosophy of ACT is one of mutuality, where the therapist is explicitly not to be considered the 'expert', that does not mean that the client will not come to feel over time like he relies upon his therapist. For this and many other reasons, the client should frequently be reminded that the therapist is fallible and human, and that the goal of therapy is to get the client out of therapy and back into his own life!

As the therapist and client begin to approach the time for termination, the work of ACT includes a more and more significant focus on reinforcing the process of values clarification and generalizing the skills of goal setting and following through on commitments in broader and broader contexts. This broadening and strengthening of the repertoire of engaging in valued behaviour is what will help the client to maintain progress, even once the therapist is no longer present. For many clients, it can be useful to ask them to generate their own list of principles that they have found to be helpful over the course of treatment, so that they have something in their own words that they can refer to when they get stuck and no longer have the therapist on which to rely. Here is one such list, generated by a very successful ACT client, and refined together with minimal assistance from the therapist. This client had stopped using substances over the course of 16 weeks of therapy and felt he was ready to begin applying ACT principles on his own:

MY 10 ACT COMMANDMENTS

1 Embrace life!
2 Fully experience my thoughts and feelings.
3 My mind will never stop, so it is useless (and sometimes even harmful) to try to control my thoughts and feelings.
4 Moods, thoughts and impulses will always change on their own – even VERY difficult ones.
5 Attempts to change thoughts and feelings will only add 'dirty' discomfort on top of the original thoughts and feelings.
6 There is NEVER a mood, thought or crisis 'bad' enough to provide a reason to use or drink.
7 Drinking or using will NEVER make a situation better!

8 I am whole and perfect, and my values need no justification.
9 I don't need to act on my thoughts or feelings or on others' expectations of me.
10 I choose to live my life in accordance with my values.

Of course, not all clients will be able to craft such an eloquent list. However, the form of such a tool is not important. What is essential is that the client has some method of retaining and integrating the information covered in therapy, so that he can continue to implement the ACT core principles throughout his life. Of note, every therapeutic modality also has some level of premature dropout from treatment, and ACT is no exception. Thus, the therapist should continually be working to reinforce a repertoire that includes generalizable principles in each session of therapy. That way, regardless of whether or not the client finishes what the therapist would judge to be a 'complete' course of treatment, he will have the foundations of a skill set that will allow him to move forward. Fortunately, several ACT studies (e.g. Gifford et al., 2004; Hayes et al., 2004a) demonstrate a pattern in which client outcomes continue to improve after termination or are better maintained over time than other treatments, even in up to 12 months follow-up. This should give therapists hope that treatment effects can persist and even grow over time when clients understand the core principles involved in behaviour change, rather than simply learning specific techniques.

As with all therapeutic challenges, some clients will have more difficulty with termination than others. For example, clients who have a significant history of interpersonal loss may have more intense feelings of sadness and anxiety (among other private events) as termination approaches. Fortunately, the general ACT model applies equally well to this situation. In such cases, the therapist raises issues of termination early and often and works with the client to accept and defuse from challenging feelings, thoughts and memories around human connection and loss. Unless the client's values include a commitment to staying in therapy forever, the therapist will work with the client on transitioning out of therapy at a pace that is consistent with the case conceptualization for each client. For some clients, this may include spacing out the final sessions with breaks in between, or leaving the possibility open for booster sessions down the road. However, it is important to remember that these methods of tapering therapeutic intervention should be done in order to support long-term skills generalization, rather than simply because it is painful for the client and therapist to say goodbye to one another.

ONGOING DEVELOPMENT AS AN ACT THERAPIST: MOVING FROM ADHERENCE TO COMPETENCE

The majority of therapists around the world choosing to learn ACT will not have the luxury of training for multiple years with an expert ACT mentor. For this reason, it is essential that interested clinicians have a basic road map for learning to implement ACT in more independent settings. Fortunately, there are now a variety of tools and methods of training for the therapist interested in learning to apply ACT principles in practice. Certainly, one of the first ways to begin to build an understanding of ACT is to read books and treatment manuals that have been developed by different authors, and a multitude of excellent references have been provided throughout this text.

Repeated presentations of the same information in different ways are more likely to lead to a nuanced understanding of the material. This applies to both written and video-based training aids. Multiple video recordings are now available (either sold together with books or ordered/ downloaded online) in which an ACT trainee can see a variety of therapists approaching similar therapeutic issues in slightly different ways. This direct modelling is especially important so that new ACT practitioners can learn to discriminate form from function in the application of ACT. By seeing that the same intervention can be delivered differently by each therapist, or that the same concept can be conveyed using totally different language, therapists learning ACT can begin to develop flexibility in implementation and find their own therapeutic 'voice'.

Similarly, for those who are able to attend ACT training workshops in person, it can be especially helpful over time to attend trainings provided by at least two different trainers. For example, one could imagine a trainee who attends an ACT workshop with a trainer who demonstrates ACT using a very specific interpersonal style. If the trainee's style is very different from that of the trainer, the trainee may think that he could never adopt that way of speaking or being in therapy. However, one can competently do ACT from a wide variety of styles – it is important not to confuse one trainer or therapist's delivery style and personality with the ACT approach itself. Thus, reading ACT texts written by a variety of authors, or attending trainings and reviewing videos in which different ACT trainers are featured, can help promote flexibility in delivery and disentangle individual trainer effects from the requirements of the therapy itself. Annual conferences of the Association for Contextual Behavioural Science provide an excellent opportunity to hear about the most recent developments in ACT from a variety of international trainers.

Although it has been stated multiple times in this volume that ACT does not need to be delivered in a rigid session-by-session format, it is recommended that those who are new to ACT do challenge themselves to work through a specific protocol in sequence several times, preferably with focused supervision, until the model is learned. The first few times that one uses a specific ACT protocol, the goal is to build adherence – the ability to correctly deliver the core ACT techniques in a planful way. Over time, with effective supervision or peer consultation, the trainee can progress from a state of pure adherence to a state of competence, in which he is more able to flexibly apply principles, techniques and meta-phors across routine and novel clinical situations. However, it is impor-tant not to skip the step of practising skills repeatedly until adherence is achieved. Otherwise, it is too easy to give in to human nature and only practise those pieces with which the therapist is already comfortable. ACT therapists are reminded that the only way to the other side of the swamp is through it, even when it comes to challenging oneself to learn new clinical skills.

One way to measure progress in adherence and competence is to use the ACT Core Competency Rating Form (Luoma et al., 2007). This sim-ple rating form can be used to assess therapist skills in the following areas: the ACT therapeutic stance, developing willingness/acceptance, undermining cognitive fusion, getting in contact with the present moment, distinguishing the conceptualized self from self-as-context, defining valued directions and building patterns of committed action. Examples of specific competences include: 'The therapist avoids the use of canned ACT interventions, instead fitting interventions to the partic-ular needs of particular clients', 'The therapist is ready to change course to fit those needs at any moment' and 'The therapist can defuse from client content and direct attention to the moment'. Depending on the resources available to the therapist, she may ask her supervisor or con-sultant to complete this form multiple times while watching or listening to recordings of the trainee therapist conducting ACT. Even if the thera-pist does not have a supervisor or consultant, she can complete the form for herself, assessing her own perceptions of her domains of strength and weakness, and identifying areas in which she could benefit from more training and practice.

Therapists wishing to learn ACT, but without access to ongoing supervision and training resources, can take heart. There is empirical evidence to support the idea that just being trained in ACT may be enough to make a clinical difference, even when the ACT therapist is not an expert and adherence and competence may not yet be fully present. For example, in an innovative clinical effectiveness study, Strosahl et al. (1998) found that providing therapists with a didactic ACT workshop and a monthly supervision group in a real-world setting was sufficient for clinical change. At the five-month follow-up point for this study, clients of those therapists who had been trained in ACT were more likely to be rated as having better levels of successful coping, were less likely to be referred for medication evaluations and were more likely to have completed therapy within five months of starting. In a further clinical effectiveness study (Lappalainen et al., 2007), trainee therapists received initial training in both CBT and ACT. Even though the therapists received limited training, the clients in the ACT condi-tion improved more with respect to both symptom improvement and the functional variable of acceptance. Thus, there are data to show that even therapists who are only able to receive a limited amount of training or supervision in ACT may be able to positively impact the functioning of their clients.

One last area for consideration of therapeutic skills acquisition involves taking the opportunity to become part of the broader ACT community. With the current state of technology, even the most remotely stationed clinician can become part of an online community of professionals who share an interest in the application of ACT around the globe. Information about online resources, including listservs and special interest groups, can be found at www.contextualpsychology.org. Many local chapters and special interest groups have been developed around the world and are associated with established professional organizations. In addition, wherever there are two interested ACT therapists who are within driving distance of one another, a local ACT peer consultation group can be formed. Such groups can function as a 'book club', serve a case consultation function or can simply provide a venue within which to problem-solve systemic implementation issues related to ACT. Truly, even locality is no longer a limiting factor, given that such consultation groups can also be created virtually, using free video-teleconferencing programmes.

FINAL CONSIDERATIONS

It may be noted that the majority of the examples provided in this text have focused on working with adults. However, the same general principles apply readily to clinical work with children and adolescents, using appropriate adaptations for cognitive maturity and developmental stages (Twohig et al., 2008; Wicksell and Greco, 2008). In fact, it could be argued that the use of metaphor and story in ACT makes this a particularly appropriate treatment modality for children.

Although ACT is already considered a highly promising clinical tool for traditional psychiatric disorders (e.g. psychosis, depression, anxiety, eating disorders), it is important to note that its reach extends beyond the realm of psychiatry into health behaviours (e.g. chronic pain, coping with illness) and more general areas of wellness and functioning (e.g. parenting, reducing stigma and prejudice). In fact, many innovative applications of ACT exist, even moving beyond the clinical setting to implementing the same principles for occupational health and organizational behaviour management (Hayes et al., 2006a).

The vision of ACT is not simply to provide an effective mechanism to achieve specific behavioural aims or clinical results, even though sufficient data exist to show that it can do so. Conveyed successfully, ACT can be a transformative approach to behaviour change that is about creating a life worth living. The ACT practitioner always keeps in mind that no client's life is hopeless. Lives can always be changed, sometimes in ways that neither the therapist nor client ever could have conceived!

ACT therapists have the honour of sitting alongside clients as they dream and aspire, and then the satisfaction of working with them as they plan, implement and transform.

Summary

The theory-driven nature of ACT is one of its most unique features. Work on six broad core processes can be brought together in a variety of ways to assist with behaviour change and improvements in life functioning. Although in-person training still provides a key method for disseminating ACT treatment skills, a variety of written, video and online training tools also exist to assist the therapist who wishes to learn ACT. Through a process of continuous practice, consultation and feedback, the clinician interested in applying ACT can move from initial interest, through adherence, and into a state of therapeutic competence in providing this innovative approach to treatment.

Points for Review and Reflection

- What might you consider when determining which ACT core process to present first in treatment?
- How should the ACT therapist approach considerations of therapy termination?
- Identify at least three ways that you can engage in ongoing learning and training in the ACT therapeutic model. How will you know if you are growing in your ACT skills and competences?

Further Reading

Bach, P.A. and Moran, D.J. (2008) *ACT in Practice: Case Conceptualization in Acceptance and Commitment Therapy*. Oakland, CA: New Harbinger Publications.

Ciarrochi, J.V. and Bailey, A. (2008) *A CBT Practitioner's Guide to ACT*. Oakland, CA: New Harbinger Publications.

Luoma, J.B., Hayes, S.C. and Walser, R.D. (2007) *Learning ACT: An Acceptance and Commitment Therapy Skills Training Manual for Therapists*. Oakland, CA: New Harbinger Publications.

Ramnero, J. and Torneke, N. (2008) *The ABCs of Human Behaviour: Behavioural Principles for the Practicing Clinician*. Oakland, CA: New Harbinger Publications.

References

Angst, F., Stassen, H.H., Clayton, P.J. and Angst, J. (2002) Mortality of patients with mood disorders: follow-up over 34–38 years. *Journal of Affective Disorders*, 68: 167–81.

Armeli, S., Tennen, H., Todd, M., Carney, M.A., Mohr, C., Affleck, G. and Hromi, A. (2003) A daily process examination of the stress-response dampening effects of alcohol consumption. *Psychology of Addictive Behaviours*, 17: 266–76.

Bach, P.A. and Hayes, S.C. (2002) The use of Acceptance and Commitment Therapy to prevent the rehospitalization of psychotic patients: a randomized controlled trial. *Journal of Consulting and Clinical Psychology*, 70: 1129–39.

Bach, P.A. and Moran, D.J. (2008) *ACT in Practice: Case Conceptualization in Acceptance and Commitment Therapy*. Oakland, CA: New Harbinger Publications.

Barlow, D.H. (2002) *Anxiety and its Disorders: The Nature and Treatment of Anxiety and Panic*, 2nd edn. New York: Guilford Press.

Batten, S.V. and Hayes, S.C. (2005) Acceptance and Commitment Therapy in the treatment of comorbid substance abuse and post-traumatic stress disorder: a case study. *Clinical Case Studies*, 4(3): 246–62.

Batten, S.V. and Santanello, A.P. (2009) A contextual behavioural approach to the role of emotion in psychotherapy supervision. *Training and Education in Professional Psychology*, 3: 148–56.

Batten, S.V., DeViva, J.C., Santanello, A.P., Morris, L.J., Benson, P.R. and Mann, M.A. (2009) Acceptance and Commitment Therapy for comorbid PTSD and substance use disorders. In J. Blackledge, J. Ciarrochi, and F. Dean (eds), *Acceptance and Commitment Therapy: Current Directions* (pp. 311–28). Queensland, Australia: Australian Academic Press.

Batten, S.V., Orsillo, S.M. and Walser, R.D. (2005) Acceptance- and mindfulness-based approaches to the treatment of posttraumatic stress disorder. In S.M. Orsillo and L. Roemer (eds), *Acceptance and Mindfulness-Based Approaches to Anxiety: Conceptualization and Treatment* (pp. 241–69). New York: Plenum Press.

Beck, A.T., Rush, A.J., Shaw, B.F. and Emery, G. (1979) *Cognitive Therapy of Depression*. New York: Guilford Press.

Block, J.A. and Wulfert, E. (2000) Acceptance or change: treating socially anxious college students with ACT or CBGT. *The Behaviour Analyst Today,* 1: 1–55.

Bonn-Miller, M.O., Vujanovic, A.A., Twohig, M.P., Medina, J.L. and Huggins, J.L. (2010) Posttraumatic stress symptom severity and marijuana use coping motives: a test of the mediating role of non-judgmental acceptance within a trauma-exposed community sample. *Mindfulness,* 1: 98–106.

Carrascoso López, F.J. (2000) Acceptance and Commitment Therapy (ACT) in panic disorder with agoraphobia: a case study. *Psychology in Spain,* 4: 120–8.

Chiles, J. and Strosahl, K. (2004) *Handbook for the Clinical Assessment and Treatment of the Suicidal Patient*. Washington, DC: American Psychiatric Press.

Ciarrochi, J.V. and Bailey, A. (2008) *A CBT Practitioner's Guide to ACT*. Oakland, CA: New Harbinger Publications.

Corrigan, P.W., River, L.P., Lundin, R.K., Wasowski, K.U., Campion, J. Mathisen, J., Goldstein, H., Bergman, M., Gagnon, C. and Kubiak, M.A. (2000) Stigmatizing attributions about mental illness. *Journal of Community Psychology,* 28: 91–102.

Dahl, J.C., Plumb, J.C., Stewart, I. and Lundgren, T. (2009) *The Art and Science of Valuing in Psychotherapy: Helping Clients Discover, Explore, and Commit to Valued Action using Acceptance and Commitment Therapy*. Oakland, CA: New Harbinger Publications.

Dalrymple, K.L. and Herbert, J.D. (2007) Acceptance and Commitment Therapy for Generalized Social Anxiety Disorder: a pilot study. *Behaviour Modification,* 31: 543–68.

Eifert, G.H. and Forsyth, J.P. (2005) *Acceptance and Commitment Therapy for Anxiety Disorders: A Practitioner's Treatment Guide to using Mindfulness, Acceptance, and Values-based Behaviour Change Strategies*. Oakland, CA: New Harbinger Publications.

Eifert, G.H., Forsyth, J.P., Arch, J., Espejo, E., Keller, M. and Langer, D. (2009) Acceptance and Commitment Therapy for anxiety disorders: three case studies exemplifying a unified treatment protocol. *Cognitive and Behavioural Practice,* 16: 368–85.

Foa, E.B. and Franklin, M.E. (2001) Obsessive-compulsive disorder. In D.H. Barlow (ed.), *Clinical Handbook of Psychological Disorders: A Step-by-Step Treatment Manual*, 3rd edn (pp. 209–63). New York: Guilford Press.

Follette, V.M. and Batten, S.V. (2000) The role of emotion in psychotherapy supervision: a contextual behavioural analysis. *Cognitive and Behavioural Practice,* 7(3): 306–12.

Follette, V.M. and Pistorello, J. (2007) *Finding Life Beyond Trauma: Using Acceptance and Commitment Therapy to Heal from Post-traumatic*

Stress and Trauma-related Problems. Oakland, CA: New Harbinger Publications.

Forman, E.M., Herbert, J.D., Moitra, E., Yeomans, P.D. and Geller, P.A. (2007) A randomized controlled effectiveness trial of Acceptance and Commitment Therapy and Cognitive Therapy for anxiety and depression. *Behaviour Modification,* 31: 772–99.

Forsyth, J.P. and Eifert, G.H. (2007) *The Mindfulness and Acceptance Workbook for Anxiety: A Guide to Breaking Free from Anxiety, Phobias and Worry using Acceptance and Commitment Therapy.* Oakland, CA: New Harbinger Publications.

Forsyth, J.P., Parker, J. and Finlay, C.G. (2003) Anxiety sensitivity, controllability, and experiential avoidance and their relation to drug of choice and addiction severity in a residential sample of substance abusing veterans. *Addictive Behaviours,* 28: 851–70.

Gaudiano, B.A. and Herbert, J.D. (2006) Acute treatment of inpatients with psychotic symptoms using Acceptance and Commitment Therapy. *Behaviour Research and Therapy,* 44: 415–37.

Gaudiano, B.A., Miller, I.W. and Herbert, J.D. (2007) The treatment of psychotic major depression: is there a role for adjunctive psychotherapy? *Psychotherapy and Psychosomatics,* 76: 271–7.

Gifford, E.V., Kohlenberg, B.S., Hayes, S.C., Antonuccio, D.O., Piasecki, M.M., Rasmussen-Hall, M.L. and Palm, K.M. (2004) Acceptance-based treatment for smoking cessation. *Behaviour Therapy,* 35: 689–705.

Glaser, N.M., Blackledge, J.T., Shepherd, L.M. and Dean, F.P. (2009) Brief group ACT for anxiety. In J. Blackledge, J. Ciarrochi and F. Dean (eds), *Acceptance and Commitment Therapy: Current Directions* (pp. 175–200). Queensland, Australia: Australian Academic Press.

Gregg, J.A., Callaghan, G.M., Hayes, S.C. and Glenn-Lawson, J.L. (2007) Improving diabetes self-management through acceptance, mindfulness, and values: a randomized controlled trial. *Journal of Consulting and Clinical Psychology,* 75(2): 336–43.

Gunaratana, H. (1992) *Mindfulness in Plain English.* Somerville, MA: Wisdom Publications.

Hanh, T.N. (1976) *The Miracle of Mindfulness.* Boston, MA: Beacon.

Harris, R. (2009) *ACT Made Simple.* Oakland, CA: New Harbinger Publications.

Hayes, S.C. (1984) Making sense of spirituality. *Behaviourism,* 12: 99–110.

Hayes, S.C. and Smith, S. (2005) *Get Out of Your Mind and Into Your Life: The New Acceptance and Commitment Therapy.* Oakland, CA: New Harbinger Publications.

Hayes, S.C., Barnes-Holmes, D. and Roche, B. (eds) (2001) *Relational Frame Theory: A Post-Skinnerian Account of Human Language and Cognition.* New York: Plenum Press.

Hayes, S.C., Bond, F.W., Barnes-Holmes, D. and Austin, J. (eds) (2006a) *Acceptance and Mindfulness at Work: Applying Acceptance and*

Commitment Therapy and Relational Frame Theory to Organizational Behaviour Management. New York: Haworth Press.

Hayes, S.C., Luoma, J.B., Bond, F.W., Masuda, A. and Lillis, J. (2006b) Acceptance and Commitment Therapy: model, processes and outcomes. *Behaviour Research and Therapy*, 44: 1–25.

Hayes, S.C., Strosahl, K.D., and Wilson, K.G. (1999) *Acceptance and Commitment Therapy: An Experiential Approach to Behaviour Change*. New York: Guilford Press.

Hayes, S.C., Wilson, K.G., Gifford, E.V., Follette, V.M. and Strosahl, K. (1996) Experiential avoidance and behavioural disorders: a functional dimensional approach to diagnosis and treatment. *Journal of Consulting and Clinical Psychology*, 64: 1152–68.

Hayes, S.C., Wilson, K.G., Gifford, E.V., Bissett, R.T., Piasecki, M., Batten, S.V., Byrd, M.R. and Gregg, J. (2004a) A preliminary trial of twelve-step facilitation and Acceptance and Commitment Therapy with polysubstance-abusing methadone-maintained opiate addicts. *Behaviour Therapy*, 35: 667–88.

Hayes, S.C., Bissett, R., Roget, N., Padilla, M., Kohlenberg, B.S., Fisher, G., Masuda, A., Pistorello, J., Rye, A.K., Berry, K. and Niccolls, R. (2004b) The impact of acceptance and commitment training and multicultural training on the stigmatizing attitudes and professional burnout of substance abuse counselors. *Behaviour Therapy*, 35: 821–35.

Hayes, S.C., Strosahl, K.D., Wilson, K.G., Bissett, R.T., Pistorello, J., Toarmino, D., Polusny, M.A., Dykstra, T.A., Batten, S.V., Bergan, J., Stewart, S.H., Zvolensky, M.J., Eifert, G.H., Bond, F.W., Forsyth J.P., Karekla, M. and McCurry, S.M. (2004c) Measuring experiential avoidance: a preliminary test of a working model. *The Psychological Record*, 54: 553–78.

Heffner, M., Eifert, G.H., Parker, B.T., Hernandez, D.H. and Sperry, J.A. (2003) Valued directions: Acceptance and Commitment Therapy in the treatment of alcohol dependence. *Cognitive and Behavioural Practice*, 10: 378–83.

Hernandez-Lopez, M., Luciano, M.C., Bricker, J.B., Roales-Nieto, J.G. and Montesinos, F. (2009) Acceptance and Commitment Therapy for smoking cessation: a preliminary study of its effectiveness in comparison with cognitive behavioural therapy. *Psychology of Addictive Behaviours*, 23: 723–30.

Kabat-Zinn, J. (1990) *Full Catastrophe Living: Using the Wisdom of Your Body and Mind to Face Stress, Pain, and Illness*. New York: Dell.

Kabat-Zinn, J. (1994) *Wherever You Go There You Are*. New York: Hyperion.

Kanter, J.W., Baruch, D.E. and Gaynor, S.T. (2006) Acceptance and Commitment Therapy and behavioural activation for the treatment of depression: description and comparison. *The Behaviour Analyst,* 29: 161–85.

Kessler, R.C., Chiu, W.T., Demler, O. and Walters, E.E. (2005) Prevalence, severity, and comorbidity of 12-month DSM-IV disorders in the National Comorbidity Survey Replication. *Archives of General Psychiatry*, 62: 617–27.

Kohlenberg, R.J. and Tsai, M. (2007) *Functional Analytic Psychotherapy: Creating Intense and Curative Therapeutic Relationships*. New York: Springer.

Lambert, M.J. and Barley, D.E. (2002) Research summary on the therapeutic relationship and psychotherapy outcome. In J.C. Norcross (ed.), *Psychotherapy Relationships that Work* (pp. 17–32). New York: Oxford University Press.

Lappalainen, R., Lehtonen, T., Skarp, E., Taubert, E., Ojanen, M. and Hayes, S.C. (2007) The impact of CBT and ACT models using psychology trainee therapists: a preliminary controlled effectiveness trial. *Behaviour Modification*, 31: 488–511.

Lindsley, O.R. (1968) Training parents and teachers to precisely manage children's behaviour. Address presented at the C.S. Mott Foundation Children's Health Center, Flint, MI, March.

Lundgren, T., Dahl, J., Melin, L. and Kies, B. (2006) Evaluation of acceptance and commitment therapy for drug refractory epilepsy: a randomized controlled trial in South Africa – a pilot study. *Epilepsia*, 47(12): 2173–9.

Luoma, J.B., Hayes, S.C. and Walser, R.D. (2007) *Learning ACT: An Acceptance and Commitment Therapy Skills Training Manual for Therapists*. Oakland, CA: New Harbinger Publications.

Luoma, J.B., Kohlenberg, B.S., Hayes, S.C., Bunting, K. and Rye, A.K. (2008) Reducing self-stigma in substance abuse through Acceptance and Commitment Therapy: model, manual development, and pilot outcomes. *Addiction Research and Theory*, 16: 149–65.

Marlatt, G.A. and Witkiewitz, K. (2005) Relapse prevention for alcohol and drug problems. In G.A. Marlatt and D.M. Donovan (eds), *Relapse Prevention: Maintenance Strategies in the Treatment of Addictive Behaviours* (pp. 1–44). New York: Guilford Press.

Martell, C.R., Addis, M.E. and Jacobson, N.S. (2001) *Depression in Context: Strategies for Guided Action*. New York: Norton.

Martell, C.R., Dimidjian, S. and Herman-Dunn, R. (2010) *Behavioural Activation for Depression: A Clinician's Guide*. New York: Guilford Press.

Murray, C.J.L. and Lopez, A.D. (eds) (1996) *The Global Burden of Disease and Injury Series, Vol. 1: A Comprehensive Assessment of Mortality and Disability from Diseases, Injuries, and Risk Factors in 1990 and Projected to 2020*. Cambridge, MA: Harvard University Press.

Narrow, W.E., Rae, D.S., Robins, L.N. and Regier, D.A. (2002) Revised prevalence estimates of mental disorders in the United States: using a clinical significance criterion to reconcile 2 surveys' estimates. *Archives of General Psychiatry*, 59: 115–23.

Norcross, J.C. (2002) Empirically supported therapy relationships. In J.C. Norcross (ed.), *Psychotherapy Relationships that Work* (pp. 3–16). New York: Oxford University Press.

Orsillo, S.M. and Batten, S.V. (2005) Acceptance and Commitment Therapy in the treatment of posttraumatic stress disorder. *Behaviour Modification*, 29(1): 95–129.

Orsillo, S.M. and Roemer, L. (in press) *The Mindful Way through Anxiety*. New York: Guilford Press.

Orsillo, S.M., Roemer, L., Block-Lerner, J., LeJeune, C. and Herbert, J.D. (2004) ACT with anxiety disorders. In S.C. Hayes and K.D. Strosahl (eds), *A Practical Guide to Acceptance and Commitment Therapy* (pp. 103–32). New York: Springer.

Petersen, C.L. and Zettle, R.D. (2009) Treating inpatients with comorbid depression and alcohol use disorders: a comparison of Acceptance and Commitment Therapy and treatment as usual. *The Psychological Record,* 59: 521–36.

Ramnero, J. and Torneke, N. (2008) *The ABCs of Human Behaviour: Behavioural Principles for the Practicing Clinician*. Oakland, CA: New Harbinger Publications.

Roemer, L. and Orsillo, S.M. (2005) An acceptance-based behaviour therapy for generalized anxiety disorder. In S.M. Orsillo and L. Roemer (eds), *Acceptance and Mindfulness-based Approaches to Anxiety: Conceptualization and Treatment* (pp. 213–40). New York: Springer.

Roemer, L., Orsillo, S.M. and Salters-Pedneault, K. (2008) Efficacy of an acceptance-based behaviour therapy for generalized anxiety disorder: evaluation in a randomized controlled trial. *Journal of Consulting and Clinical Psychology,* 76: 1083–9.

Ruiz, F.J. (2010) A review of Acceptance and Commitment Therapy (ACT) empirical evidence: correlational, experimental psychopathology, component and outcome studies. *International Journal of Psychology and Psychological Therapy*, 10: 125–62.

Stewart, S.H. and Zeitlin, S.B. (1995) Anxiety sensitivity and alcohol use motives. *Journal of Anxiety Disorders*, 9: 229–40.

Stotts, A.L., Masuda, A. and Wilson, K. (2009) Using Acceptance and Commitment Therapy during methadone dose reduction: rationale, treatment, description, and a case report. *Cognitive and Behavioral Practice*, 16: 205–13.

Strosahl, K.D. (2004) ACT with the multi-problem patient. In S.C. Hayes and K.D. Strosahl (eds), *A Practical Guide to Acceptance and Commitment Therapy* (pp. 209–45). New York: Springer.

Strosahl, K.D. and Robinson, P.J. (2008) *The Mindfulness and Acceptance Workbook for Depression: Using Acceptance and Commitment Therapy to Move through Depression and Create a Life Worth Living*. Oakland, CA: New Harbinger Publications.

Strosahl, K.D., Hayes, S.C., Bergan, J. and Romano, P. (1998) Assessing the field effectiveness of Acceptance and Commitment Therapy: an example of the manipulated training research method. *Behaviour Therapy*, 29: 35–64.

Titchener, E.B. (1916) *A Textbook of Psychology*. New York: Macmillan.

Twohig, M.P. (2008) *ACT Verbatim for Depression and Anxiety*. Oakland, CA: New Harbinger Publications.

Twohig, M.P. (2009a) Acceptance and Commitment Therapy for treatment-resistant posttraumatic stress disorder: a case study. *Cognitive and Behavioural Practice*, 16: 243–52.

Twohig, M.P. (2009b) The application of Acceptance and Commitment Therapy to obsessive-compulsive disorder. *Cognitive and Behavioural Practice*, 16: 18–28.

Twohig, M.P., Hayes, S.C. and Berlin, K.S. (2008) Acceptance and Commitment Therapy for childhood externalizing disorders. In L.A. Greco and S.C. Hayes (eds), *Acceptance and Mindfulness Treatments for Children and Adolescents: A Practitioner's Guide* (pp. 163–86). Oakland, CA: New Harbinger Press.

Twohig, M.P., Hayes, S.C. and Masuda, A. (2006) Increasing willingness to experience obsessions: Acceptance and Commitment Therapy as a treatment for obsessive-compulsive disorder. *Behaviour Therapy*, 37: 3–13.

Twohig, M.P., Shoenberger, D. and Hayes, S.C. (2007) A preliminary investigation of Acceptance and Commitment Therapy as a treatment for marijuana dependence in adults. *Journal of Applied Behaviour Analysis*, 40: 619–32.

Walser, R.D. and Westrup, D. (2007) *Acceptance and Commitment Therapy for the Treatment of Post-traumatic Stress Disorder and Trauma Related Problems*. Oakland, CA: New Harbinger Publications.

Wicksell, R.K. and Greco, L.A. (2008) Acceptance and Commitment Therapy for pediatric chronic pain. In L.A. Greco and S.C. Hayes (eds), *Acceptance and Mindfulness Treatments for Children and Adolescents: A Practitioner's Guide* (pp. 89–113). Oakland, CA: New Harbinger Press.

Wicksell, R.K., Ahlqvist, J., Bring, A., Melin, L. and Olsson, G.L. (2008) Can exposure and acceptance strategies improve functioning and life satisfaction in people with chronic pain and whiplash-associated disorders (WAD)? A randomized controlled trial. *Cognitive Behaviour Therapy*, 37(3): 1–14.

Wicksell, R.K., Melin, L., Lekander, M. and Olsson, G.L. (2009) Evaluating the effectiveness of exposure and acceptance strategies to improve functioning and quality of life in longstanding pediatric pain – a randomized controlled trial. *Pain*, 141(3): 248–57.

Williams, L.M. (2007) Acceptance and Commitment Therapy: an example of third-wave therapy as a treatment for Australian Vietnam War veterans with posttraumatic stress disorder (PTSD). *Salute*, 19: 13–15.

Williams, M., Teasdale, J., Segal, Z. and Kabat-Zinn, J. (2007) *The Mindful Way through Depression: Freeing Yourself from Chronic Unhappiness*. New York: Guilford Press.

Wilson, K.G. and Byrd, M.R. (2004) ACT for substance abuse and dependence. In S.C. Hayes and K.D. Strosahl (eds), *A Practical Guide to Acceptance and Commitment Therapy* (pp. 153–84). New York: Springer.

Wilson, K.G. and Dufrene, T. (2008) *Mindfulness for Two: An Acceptance and Commitment Therapy Approach to Mindfulness in Psychotherapy.* Oakland, CA: New Harbinger Publications.

Wilson, K.G. and Sandoz, E.K. (2008) Mindfulness, values and therapeutic relationship in Acceptance and Commitment Therapy. In S.F. Hick and T. Bien (eds), *Mindfulness and the Therapeutic Relationship* (pp. 89–106). New York: Guilford Press.

Wilson, K.G., Hayes, S.C. and Byrd, M.R. (2000) Exploring compatibilities between Acceptance and Commitment Therapy and 12-step treatment for substance abuse. *Journal of Rational-Emotive Behaviour Therapy*, 18: 209–34.

Zettle, R.D. (2004) ACT with affective disorders. In S.C. Hayes and K.D. Strosahl (eds), *A Practical Guide to Acceptance and Commitment Therapy* (pp. 77–102). New York: Springer.

Zettle, R.D. (2007) *ACT for Depression: A Clinician's Guide to Using Acceptance and Commitment Therapy in Treating Depression.* Oakland, CA: New Harbinger Publications.

Zettle, R.D. and Hayes, S.C. (1986) Dysfunctional control by client verbal behaviour: the context of reason giving. *The Analysis of Verbal Behaviour,* 4: 30–8.

Zettle, R.D. and Rains, J.C. (1989) Group cognitive and contextual therapies in treatment of depression. *Journal of Clinical Psychology*, 45: 436–45.

Zettle, R.D., Barner, S.L. and Gird, S. (2009) ACT with depression: the role of forgiving. In J. Blackledge, J. Ciarrochi and F. Dean (eds), *Acceptance and Commitment Therapy: Current Directions* (pp. 151–73). Queensland, Australia: Australian Academic Press.

Zettle, R.D., Rains, J.C. and Hayes, S.C. (in press) Processes of change in Acceptance and Commitment Therapy and cognitive therapy for depression: a mediational reanalysis of Zettle and Rains (1989). *Behaviour Modification.*

Index

ACBS, *see* Association for Contextual Behavioral Science
Acceptance, 12, 23–6, 78, 101, 113
Actions, 25, 58, 66–73, 92, 103, 109
Addictive disorders, 103–15
Adherence and competence, 7, 111–15
Agoraphobia, 3, 31, 79
Alcohol use, *see* Substance abuse/misuse
Alexithymia, 16
Anhedonia, 86
Anxiety, 3, 6, 19, 21, 26, 34, 67, 75–84, 88, 95, 111
  conceptualization of, 21, 75–7, 80–2
Assessment, 61, 67, 91, 96–7, 107–8
Association for Contextual Behavioral Science, 112
Avoidance, 1–3, 6–8, 10, 14–5, 21–3, 25, 27, 42, 53, 57, 61, 63, 66–7, 76–83, 86, 95–8, 100, 102, 104, 107–9
Awareness, 13, 16, 22, 35–45, 52, 77, 88

Barriers, 14, 45, 66–73, 82, 92, 109
Behavioural activation, 85, 92–3
Bicycle metaphor, 11, 24, 30, 71–2
Boundaries, 9, 14, 16
Breathing, 24, 39–40, 62, 77–8, 101

Case conceptualization, 1–2, 27, 39, 44, 53, 63, 75–6, 81, 86, 90, 102, 107–9, 111
CBT, *see* Cognitive behavioural therapy
Chessboard metaphor, 51–2
Children, 47, 114
Chronic pain, 5, 114
Cigarettes, *see* Smoking
Clouds in the sky, 40–1, 52
Cognitive behavioural therapy, 6, 32, 36, 66, 75, 77, 83, 85–6, 96, 113
Cognitive fusion, *see* Fusion
Commitment, 66–73, 87, 90, 100–2, 110
Committed action, 3, 64, 66–73, 80, 90, 92, 95, 102, 107, 109, 113
Competence, 105, 111–14
  assessment of, 113

Conceptualized self, 2, 47–8, 52, 54, 88–90, 113
Consultation, peer, 15, 63, 105, 112, 114–15
Contact with the present, 37–45, 49, 57, 64, 66, 77, 88, 93, 95, 100–1, 104, 107, 113
Container with stuff in it, 51, 54
Context, 9–10, 14, 16, 22, 26, 28, 35–7, 43–4, 49, 51, 60, 63, 90, 98, 110
Contextualism, 1, 7, 37, 105
Contextualpsychology.org, 61, 71, 107, 114
Control, 60, 76, 78, 83, 91, 99
  as the problem, 18–27, 77, 98, 110
Creative hopelessness, 20–3, 27, 63, 76–7, 97, 108

Defusion, 13, 28–30, 32–7, 42, 45, 49, 63, 66, 69, 72, 77–8, 80, 83, 86–8, 91–3, 105, 107
Deliteralization, *see* Defusion
Depression, 3, 5–6, 20–1, 32, 46, 85–95, 102, 114
Desert Island, 58–9

Emotion, 12, 15–16, 29, 45, 54, 61, 69, 91, 109
Eulogy, 58–9
Experiential avoidance, *see* Avoidance
Expert, 9–10, 16, 69, 106, 110–1, 113
Exposure, 5, 67, 75, 77–8, 80–3
Exposure exercises, *see* Exposure
Eyes closed, 44, 53, 58

Flexibility, psychological, 2–3, 13, 18, 28, 34, 37, 45, 48, 62, 67, 75, 77–8, 83, 90, 108, 112–13
Forgiveness, 92–3
Functional analysis, 2, 86, 90, 97, 108
Fusion, 2–4, 7, 10, 28–36, 42, 66, 76, 82–3, 86, 108–9, 113

GAD, *see* Generalized anxiety disorder
Gardening, 68
Generalization of skills, 43–5, 110–111
Generalized anxiety disorder, 79, 82

Goals, 15, 56–8, 62, 64, 66–73, 90, 95,
    100–2, 108
  dead man's, 68
  of ACT, 21, 28–9, 32, 34–6, 48–9, 52, 61,
    67, 89, 91–3, 102, 110
Grief, 88–9
Group therapy, 42, 71, 82, 84, 87, 98

House with furniture in it, 50–1
Humour, *see* Irreverence

Ice meditation, *see* Mindfulness on the rocks
Informed consent, 19
Invalidating, *see* Validation
Irreverence, 12–13, 33, 35, 75

Language, 4, 28–37, 47, 86–7, 98
  conventions, 33–6, 87
Leaves in the stream, 41
Life Story exercise, 88–90, 93
Literality, 28–31, 34–5, 48, 77

Memorial service, 58–9
Metaphors, role of, 4, 15, 21, 24–6, 33, 58, 64,
    72, 77, 106, 109, 114
Milk, milk, milk, 31–2, 77
Mind, 4, 28–34, 41–2, 47, 52, 77, 91, 110
Mindfulness, 3, 12–13, 32, 35, 37–46, 49–50,
    52–3, 56, 63, 68–70, 72, 77, 82, 88, 91–2,
    100–1, 104, 110
  of breathing, 39–40, 42
  of five senses, 41–3, 53
  of music, 41, 43
Mindfulness on the rocks, 42–3

Notecards, 24, 26, 29, 32

Observer exercise, 50
Observing self, 48–54
Obsessive-compulsive disorder, 75, 79–81
OCD, *see* Obsessive-compulsive disorder

Panic, 3, 24, 26, 75–7, 79–81
Parenting, 60, 114
Pausing in the moment, 70, 101
Pliance, 62, 64, 69, 71
Post-traumatic stress disorder, 3, 6, 75, 78–9,
    81, 99, 102, 104
Power differential, 10–11
Pragmatism, 1, 7, 105–6
Progressive self questions, 49–50, 53
Psychotic disorders, 5–6, 87, 114
PTSD, *see* Post-traumatic stress disorder

Quicksand, 20–3, 26, 76

Relational frame theory, 4, 8
Rescuing, 13, 71
Respect, 12–13, 16, 19, 64, 97, 106
RFT, *see* Relational frame theory
Rule-governed behaviour, 4, 7, 14, 34–5, 38,
    61–4, 71

Self, 2, 34, 47–55, 81, 86, 88–90, 113
Self-as-content, *see* Conceptualized self
Self-as-context, 2, 37, 47–55, 63, 66, 80, 92–3,
    105, 107, 113
Self-disclosure, 15
Sense of self, 48–9, 81
Senses, five, 41–3, 53
Smoking, 6, 96, 99–101, 103
Substance abuse/misuse, 3, 6, 21, 23, 38, 57,
    95–104, 112
Substance use disorders, *see* Substance
    abuse/misuse
Suicidal behaviour, 3, 6, 85, 90–3
Suicide, 90–2
Supervision, 12, 15–17, 112–14
Swallowing, 62
Swamp, 26, 31, 63, 113

Termination, 110–11, 115
Theory, importance of, 1, 4, 105–6, 115
Therapeutic relationship, 2, 9–17, 33, 35, 93,
    96, 103
Therapist, in the same boat, 10–11
Tombstone, 59
Trauma history, 4, 15, 44, 53, 57, 81
Twelve steps, 99, 103–4, 119
Two mountains, 11, 72

Validation, 10–12, 15, 19, 32, 35, 53, 64, 72,
    92–3
Valued life directions, *see* Values
Values, 1–2, 7, 10, 12–13, 15–16, 18, 25,
    27–8, 34–5, 37–8, 45, 48, 52, 54,
    56–75, 78, 80–3, 90–3, 95, 97, 100–7,
    108–11, 113
  assessment of, 62, 67, 97, 107
  conflicts in, 62–3
  domains of, 3, 60–2, 64, 67–8, 97

Willingness, 18–27, 30, 42, 63–4, 66, 69, 72,
    76, 78, 80–3, 86, 88, 91–3, 96–8, 103,
    109, 113
Workability, 13–14, 16, 22, 25–6, 28, 34–5,
    56, 63, 86, 91, 93, 96–8, 103, 105–6

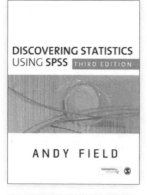
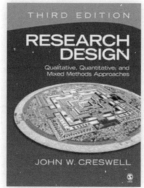
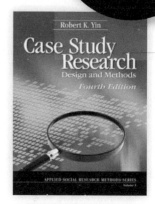
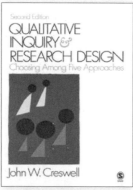
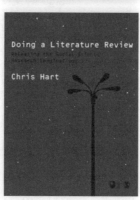
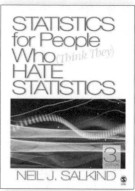
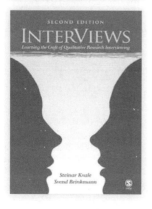
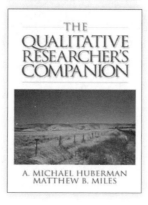
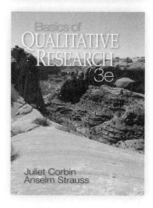
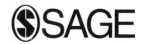